RECOVERY 2-DAY™

NORTH PASS

TELEMACHUS
PRESS
N
W — ◇ — E
S

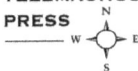

WARNING AND DISCLAIMER: The Recovery 2-Day™ Program is presented as a suggested treatment plan that teaches techniques and methods used to improve one's health. All information relating to medical conditions, health issues, products, and treatments are not meant to be a substitute for the advice of your own physician or other medical professional. You should not use the information herein to diagnose or treat yourself and should consult with your physician or medical professional before making changes to any medications or doctor recommended treatment programs of any kind. Although this program has been designed with recovery in mind, the recovery period for each individual may vary, as personal recovery is subjective and the results cannot be guaranteed because recovery for any one person or persons progresses in various stages. It is recognized that the Recovery 2-Day™ methods are to be used voluntarily and that the Recovery 2-Day™ Program and its representatives are to be held harmless from any persons or organizations using its methods.

Cover Art Design: Telemachus Press, LLC
Illustrations:
   Copyright © istockphoto.com/Sophia Tsibikaki (Trapped Man)
   Copyright © istockphoto.com/Andrew Parfenov (Gravestone)
   Copyright © istockphoto.com/art12321 8704698
   Copyright © istockphoto.com/cyrop 575103
   Copyright © istockphoto.com/Eliza Snow 10330989
   Copyright © istockphoto.com/David Ciemny 4587940
   Copyright © istockphoto.com/Bartosz Hadyniak 11441231
   Copyright © istockphoto.com/porcorex 10583936
   Copyright © istockphoto.com/geopaul 5773171
   Copyright © istockphoto.com/Grafissimo 591203
   Copyright © istockphoto.com/Mark Stay 7482401
   Copyright © istockphoto.com/Adriana Rodarte 3978192
   Copyright © istockphoto.com/Gregory Spencer 2444497
   Copyright © istockphoto.com/dmcmurdie 11673154
   Copyright © istockphoto.com/Leo Blanchette 4446884
   Copyright © istockphoto.com/Palto 9393836
   Copyright © istockphoto.com/ktsimage 3541361, 3598748, 3828878
   5192992, 3590577, 3772632, 7246931, 9392030, 3601792
   4178578, 5152985

ISBN: 978-1-935670-13-1 (North Pass Edition Paperback)
ISBN: 978-1-935670-14-8 (South Pass Edition Paperback)
ISBN: 978-1-935670-20-9 (Combined North and South Pass Editions)

Visit the author website: http://www.recovery2day.org

Published by: Telemachus Press, LLC – http://www.telemachuspress.com

Learn it in a day.
Practice it for a lifetime.

AVOIDING THE READ AROUND

Recovery 2-Day™ makes every effort to avoid debates and obstacles that cause a person to reject a treatment plan, because *words matter*.

We have a unique way of dealing with this. Recovery 2-Day™ gives each individual the respect they deserve by not making someone read around words that might block them from seeking help. Certain words affect people's ability to participate in their own recovery. We respect the differences, rather than forcing someone to convert to ours. This means the person holding this book and having a different belief than the next person can choose either the South or North Pass text, or the edition that contains both passes.

This NORTH PASS EDITION
Does not contains tools that use terms like God, prayer, etc.

Choice based in belief, Recovery 2-Day™ supplies the way for a person to select their own recovery tools instead of being forced to fit into a one size-fits-all approach. You have entered the hallway of your choice.

PREFACE

Recovery 2-Day™ begins with an apology.
We are so very sorry this has happened to you.

The reason we offer this apology to you now and throughout the book is that we mean it. Many people have battled substance abuse and dependence for years, and yet the majority of the world dismisses them as one of those, instead of regarding them as normal human beings who are battling a problem with a potential disease. We feel an apology is needed and long overdue.

Now, let us tell you how you are going to benefit from Recovery 2-Day™.

You might have come to a time or place in your life when a substance, it does not matter what it is, has caused you to ask yourself, *Should I quit?* Perhaps you tried to quit on your own and found that you needed help. The natural question that follows is, *Where can I go for help?*

If a person has a serious problem, such as substance abuse, we believe that it makes sense they seek answers from those who have lived through the same experience. They need to seek out guides who can honestly state, *We quit and stayed quit. And this is how we did it.*

Recovery 2-Day™ is a complete recovery treatment plan, beginning at day zero when you first enter into Recovery 2-Day™ until the moment you decide you can finish the course on your own. Recovery 2-Day™ is designed to be open-ended. It is intended to remove every obstacle that prevents you from staying substance-free for the rest of your life. Our goal is to help you arrive safely on the other side of your substance-abuse problem. It's a healthy, practical, common sense approach – it is not a belief system and does not reside in any form of ideology. You don't have to buy into anything or sign up for anything. All we offer are practical methods that will help you achieve permanent abstinence. Not only that, though: You will achieve much more than just not using a substance. Our tools are developed for the purpose of showing you how you can live a healthy, happy, fulfilled life, not just how to abstain. You will actually get well in all areas of your life.

We need two things from you, your trust and your hope.

There are an estimated 20.8 million people in the United States alone who have a substance abuse problem. Research in this recovery industry is ongoing, but the current research focuses mostly on the damaging effects of substance abuse on the human brain. The research covers both short and long term exposure to a substance that is foreign to our human organism. The medical and science studies show the human brain before, during, and after exposure to drugs or alcohol. The findings are critical to the effective methods and techniques unique to Recovery 2-Day™. For example, one of the first tools we offer is called the Stroop Chart, a powerful psychological tool used to interrupt cravings.

Recovery 2-Day™ was developed to bring new and successful information to the men and women who need it the most, including anyone having a substance problem.

What determines abuse from dependence? In other words, how do you answer the first question that needs to be addressed: *Do I have a problem?*

Only you can answer that question, no one else. But you need to have a picture of the difference between having a problem and not having a problem. Carlton K. Erickson, Ph.D. describes the difference as *Grim* and *Grave*. Abuse or misuse is *Grim*. Chemical dependence is *Grave*.

This is important, since you may have a preconceived image in your mind of what an alcoholic or drug addict looks like.

You might be surprised. They look like anyone else. There are, as we said earlier, twenty million substance abusers in the United States alone. They might look just like you do.

If you have come to that place and time in your life when you say to yourself: *I think I do*, or *I am afraid I do*, what are you going to do about it?

Age, race, and gender make no difference. There is no protection in believing that you are too young, or too old, or too beautiful, or too smart.

You may have been told it is a disease, and in some ways this is true. Substance dependence can lead to the disease of addiction, and this is a complex problem.

But, simply put, if you follow the practical methods and techniques that we offer here in our Recovery 2-Day™ program, you will get well. It may take some time, and it certainly takes a strong commitment, **but you will get well.**

Everyone is welcome in Recovery 2-Day™. We do not label you with industry terms such as addict or alcoholic but simply use the uniform word 'substance' that covers all addictions. Labels or self-descriptors create a long-term negative reinforcement or stigma, so we have removed them.

We treat you with the respect you deserve. You were given a name at birth, and that is the only appropriate label that should be used.

On your entry into the Recovery 2-Day™ we used the metaphor of climbing a mountain. We chose Mt Everest since it has two sides that most people choose to climb when they make the ascent: either the North Pass or the South Pass. Mt. Everest is the highest peak on our planet. Men, women, and children have all climbed it successfully, but it is not easy. The peak challenges them all.

Depending on the book you have, you may be reading a North Pass or South Pass Edition. Or you may have a book that appears to have 2 front covers, depending on which way you turn the book (inverted).We created two passes or methods/techniques for anyone to practice. You start to see the number 2, of our name Recovery 2 Day™, begins to represent many twos.

The two passes represent your personal beliefs. We respect your choice.

The world is comprised of two basic groups, those who believe in spirituality and those who do not. We use the terms religious, religion and spirituality synonymously, in their broadest, most inclusive of meanings, ranging from affiliated, unaffiliated, new age, spiritual, to conventional or church-going. We know that agnostics and atheists have very strong beliefs and needed to be treated with the same respect. The aim of recovery shifts from *belief based* to *results based*, while honoring each personal belief. Who or how you worship is not our concern, and if groups of people have different beliefs, this again, is none of our business. We accept the fact that the world holds different beliefs. The question becomes, *How does Recovery 2 Day™ create a hallway to bridge where we can create safe boundaries for all the different beliefs where we need them?* We will use the important spiritual tools of prayer and meditation that have been developed by spiritual bodies, as much as we use tools developed by science or medical professionals. In Recovery 2 Day we have married science, cognitive therapy techniques, religion, medical and common sense in a practice that will help anyone with a substance misuse or dependence problem, and which avoids all the obstacles that might prevent a person from getting the help they need.

By adopting the medical criteria of substance abuse and dependence, we removed the social stigma and moral question. The problem itself is secular. Alcohol or drugs do not care if you are a Christian, Jew, Muslim, Hindu, Buddhist, agnostic or atheist, and they care nothing about your age, race, and gender.

The problem of alcoholism or addiction is completely fair in its destruction and affects both those who pray and those who do not. It also is considered the first truly equal opportunity employer of its kind. We can say it loved us when no one else would. It is difficult to leave such a love, even when it harshly turns on us like an unrequited love.

Our solution to the problem of belief systems is to eliminate the debate by creating two methods to honor all beliefs.

So if you have a religious belief, use one set of tools. If you don't have religious beliefs, use a different set of tools. This is the reason for the inverted book.

Both groups get well!

Agnostics and atheists in many self-help groups traditionally have been forced to accept a god instead of having a program respecting their beliefs. Historically, they have never been given a choice. For years, the approach has been: "Do this or leave." We see the leave part as signing a death certificate for many.

The beauty of using the medical model as prescribed by the American Medical Association (AMA) and American Psychiatric Association (APA) is the problem is a secular one, not a moral issue. We have eliminated the need for separation and combined the addict and alcoholic. We dropped the terms and called them both substances, and this means both groups are welcome. The tools designed to treat a substance are the exact same tools for a person with a prescription, street drug or alcohol problem. The substance does not matter.

By ending the need to adapt or leave, based in faith, religions, and religious practices, and by creating 2 passes, this never forces anyone to adapt or adapt to our personal beliefs.

No one is left standing on the outside looking in. You are welcome here, no matter what substance you use, or how much, or what you believe, or whether you believe at all.

This is the goal of Recovery 2-Day™

**We truly unite and invite
all men and women to get well,
2-Day.**

WE UNDERSTAND

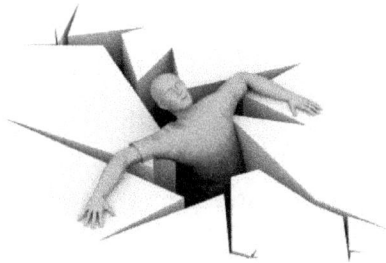

We understand that since you are reading this book the chances are good you do not want to be in this position. You may or may not even agree you have a problem, and perhaps you are here simply because someone else thinks you have a problem. We often believe someone else is at fault for the situation we are in, rather than it being anything we have done. We are even prepared to prove it, if only someone would listen.

Perhaps someone in your family or a good friend believes you have a problem. Or a judge, legal system or employer also believes you have a problem. Perhaps a medical board or treatment professional person believes you have a problem. So here you are, sitting in your home or in a room full of strangers, dazed, angry, and confused, not sure whether you have a problem, and you are trying to explain to strangers the reasons you should not be here. You may already know you have a problem, but you continue to believe no one can or will understand you. Maybe you believe that others are responsible. Everyone would understand your situation, if they only knew your childhood, your parents, the relationships you had, your neighborhood, your job, your debt, or your fear of someone finding out your secret.

While reading this book or attending meetings, you will hear others speaking openly of their problems with substance abuse or substance dependence, depending on the type of meeting you have to attend. Often the conversations are about things you had hoped no one would ever know about you. Sometimes this open sharing seems like someone has been spying on your life, and it feels like your privacy has been invaded. You may have lived through years of shame and never wanted the truth to be revealed. The idea of speaking about it openly with strangers is unthinkable.

If you knew what I had done, you would not sit next to me.

This is exactly the type of intimate talk a person who has suffered either substance abuse or substance dependence, or both, would understand. The healing power of one sufferer to another is beyond our comprehension, but there is healing power in hearing the words, "I know; me too."

However, there must be more than compassionate understanding. This is why trust and hope are necessary to move forward.

Trust describes it best. Hearing the words "I know; me too" spoken by someone else after years of believing that no one would understand does something for you. It helps to move you and to allow you a second look around. Who are these people?

Feeling forced into something terrifying almost seems insane. The very idea of being forced into recovery by a family member, judge, employer, or men and women of the professional medical assembly feels almost like a death sentence. It means giving up control, or what we believe is control.

So you've arrived feeling conflicted, asking, *Who am I, what's wrong,* and *how am I ever going to get out of all this trouble?*

No one likes to be told what to do. But is this really the case? Have not drugs, alcohol, or both dictated why you are sitting here today?

Say someone has sentenced you or forced you to attend recovery meetings. Hearing a family member threatening to leave is as powerful as a judge threatening a prison sentence. How you have arrived here is really the same, whether a judge, family member, medical professional gave the order or you simply came to in a moment of clarity and realized that you needed help. You may have court papers needing to be signed, or you may have family or friends dropping you off in the parking lot. You may have a terrible fear of returning to that night in the past. Everyone is, in some way, forced through these doors.

Now look around you and you will see a different stranger. They, like you, have also been forced here. Nobody really wants to be here, so you can start to relax.

It is too soon to ask you this question: *Hasn't something gone terribly wrong?* First we have to gain your trust. We simply want to establish at this point the various ways men and women arrive and move cautiously ahead.

What about the judge who sentenced you to attend some time period in meetings rather than time in jail? Did the sentence seem fair? Are you not free to do what you want to do? The answer is no. Certain laws are made to protect us from ourselves. This is why you will hear from certain members saying they are indebted to or grateful for the men and women dressed in black robes. These authorities sentenced them to seek help in Recovery 2-Day™ (R2D). They accepted Recovery 2-Day™'s help and got well.

Yes, some coming to Recovery 2-Day™ and hearing the stories shared by others might say, "I'm not that bad. I have not lost my family. I have not lost my job. I have not lost anything. Why are you bothering me? I can quit anytime I want!" And they really believe it. To them we reply, "That may be true." It is not true for most of us, but all of us, at one time or another, believed that same thing. Here at Recovery 2-Day™ we say that you have a problem when you say to yourself, "Yes, I have a problem," or even "Maybe I have a problem.: That statement is an indication you may want help.

We understand how uncomfortable it feels to be told you have a problem with drugs, alcohol, or both.

What if it is true? What now? Why trust anyone? Is there anyone to trust? Many people in the early stages of recovery repeat to themselves: "Those people do not look like me. They do not talk like me. They cannot possibly understand me, and they will not like me if I tell them the things I do or have done in the past."

If you are one of them, pause here and ask yourself this: *What did I dream of becoming when I was a child?* Has something gone terribly wrong? Have you just walked out of a crack house? Walked away from a car accident? Walked out of a twenty-year marriage? Have you lost a business, your family, or are you in the process of losing it all? Did a doctor say you are going to die? Or did you wake up one morning and say, *never again?*

What if the people who sent you to Recovery 2-Day™ are right? What if you do have a problem? Is it possible to escape from drug addiction? From alcoholism? What would life be like without drugs or alcohol?

Would you like to find out? Are you ready? Can you trust us? We hope that you will, since we have been where you are. And we can look you in your eyes, and tell you, we do not live that way anymore, and **you don't have to either.**

There is another kind of person who shows up at Recovery 2-Day™, and perhaps this is you. We call this other type a *walk in customer*. This person realized they had a problem all on their own. They are very easy to help, since there is no immediate resistance to accepting help, so if you are one of them, we're glad you're here. You realized you were in trouble, and sought help for their problem. This moment of harsh clarity and self-admission is painful no matter how you arrive in Recovery 2-Day™, and we congratulate you on your courage and determination.

VISUAL AIDS THAT
INTERRUPT CRAVINGS

The idea of quitting can make you extremely nervous. The first hurdle you have to face is craving. Craving creates the mental obsession and emotional stress of life without the substance our bodies have grown used to and expect. While detoxing, you experience various symptoms, ranging from mild obsession to the idea of *This feels impossible*.

To help you in these first critical days, we introduce three tools to use while you read the rest of our treatment plan and start to incorporate Recovery 2-Day™ into to your daily regime of getting well.

In this section, we offer you three very effective tools to help you break your habit of craving:

The Stroop Chart, the Eye Movement Desensitization and Reprocessing (EMDR) technique, and another visual aid, the Stop Sign.

Each tool can be used in conjunction with the other, each has different directions.

THE STROOP CHART
(The Book Cover)

One of the most effective methods to break your habit of craving is something called the Stroop Chart.

The Stroop Chart, developed by John Ridley Stroop, is a powerful psychological tool from the middle 1930's, used today in cognitive psychology. The Stroop Effect is created by reading the ink color aloud on a simple chart. Our memories are interrupted by a conflict of sorts that our senses (eyes) see, compared to what is stored in our memories, which causes a natural interruption.

You'll find the Stroop Chart on our book cover. As you see, it is a visual mental craving interrupter tool. By using the Stroop chart, you'll create the Stroop Effect, a sensory memory process that is interrupted. By using it, you'll break or interrupt your emotional-memory that lives in the sensation called craving. First, we need to show our brains a stored memory event. This simple chart shows us rationally how we see or sense memory. The brain can run a different process than the one it is used to, in our case using at the onset of craving. By the term using, we mean returning to the substance we abused or became dependent on.

This simple-looking chart can interrupt your cravings. We ask that in your early days you use this at least four times a day. It will show your brain how to change its memory/mind. We mentioned cognitive thought processes in the preface. This Stroop chart will show you how a mental process works, showing how stored emotion-memory will rule automatically and follow a process. Stored memory, short-term memory or long-term memory is a process we rely on. But what happens when we stored the memory and now need our cognitive thinking and reasoning, to make a decision? What happens to memory if it was encoded incorrectly when it was being encoded or stored into our brains? Being high while storing memory will filter all that memory with an "I was high" memory, stored as my truth, but it is still flawed. What happened if we encoded some memory while our brains were still developing, since development does not stop until the age of twenty-five or twenty-six? Common sense tells us it is possible we have flawed memories, sometimes referred to as euphoric recall. We remember the fun stuff, not the truth or details of what really happened. However, it will be your truth since is it your memory being used in the daily decisions.

The Stroop chart demonstrates how this memory process works. It will show a basic stored memory and how to stop or interrupt a conflict between what you see (the words), and what is actually being seen (the color).

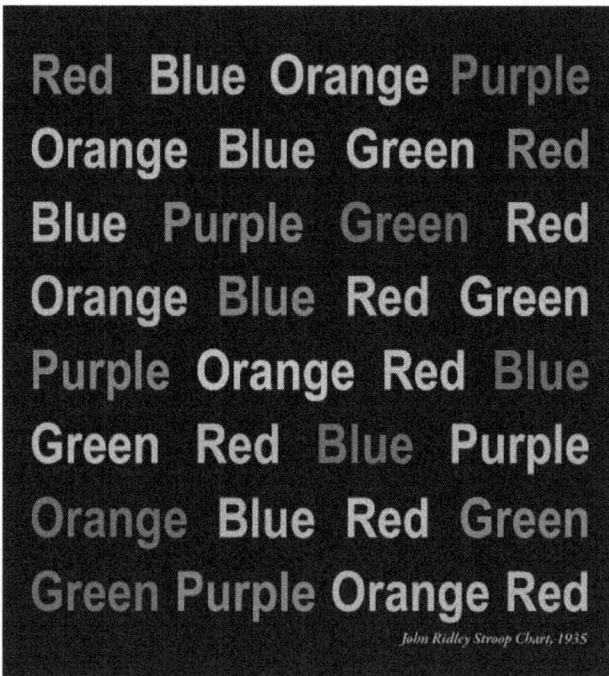

Red Blue Orange Purple
Orange Blue Green Red
Blue Purple Green Red
Orange Blue Red Green
Purple Orange Red Blue
Green Red Blue Purple
Orange Blue Red Green
Green Purple Orange Red

John Ridley Stroop Chart, 1935

When a craving event occurs, look at the book's cover. Use these directions:

First, read the words on the book cover from left to right, top to bottom quickly. Then return to the top, read from left to right calling out the color of the ink. Example: The ink color of the first word is red. The ink color of the second word is s.

Now call out the color of the ink for the remaining words. Try to go as fast as you can. When you do this, you will feel the difference. You will go slower and probably make a mistake or two. This is called the Stroop Effect.

Do this four times a day, and you will see a marked difference in cravings. It disarms or disables the craving. This is how you undo a thought process. Storing memory in the brain is a sensory process. If it is encoded correctly, it works wonderfully. If it is encoded (remembered-sensed) incorrectly, the results are predictable.

Our website www.recovery2day.org offers multiple Stroop Charts free to download.

EYE MOVEMENT
DESENSITIZATION
AND REPROCESSING (EMDR)

Another method for interrupting craving is called Eye Movement Desensitization and Reprocessing (EMDR) developed by Francine Shapiro, PhD in 1989. Mainly used in the treatment of Post-Traumatic Stress Disorder (PTSD) patients, this tool can also be effective with certain men and women. It has to do with having certain memories locked in, such as a craving memory or trauma event. To break or interrupt the cravings try this simple method.

Close your eyes. While closed, move your eyes hard left, then hard right then hard left and hard right again. Do this three times with your eyes closed. It takes only seconds to do this.

This does not work with all people. However, some it does affect are released from the distressed memories that only moments ago were non-stop, allowing a person temporarily to unlock from the locked traumatic memory. Most people are visual in their memories. By closing the eyes and moving them while closed, this seems to break the process of the past visual association.

STOP

Another effective method we have used to help you if you're experiencing physical cravings in the early days of Recovery 2-Day™ is a simple stop sign.

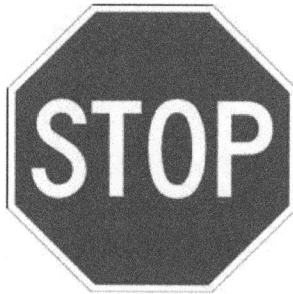

This is a universal sign. It means stop. Most people, no matter how destitute they are, have a cell phone in today's society. Take a picture of a street stop sign and set it as the screen saver on your cell phone. In group, we use this visually as group meditation practice. Close your eyes, relax, breathe in, exhale, breathe in, exhale, now visually bring forth the image of a stop sign in your mind's eye. Breathe in, exhale, relax, open your eyes.

This simple but effective visual aid has calmed many a mind's eye while craving.

These are three simple yet very effective tools that you can use in your first days of recovery. Now we can move on to the daily life once you're firmly in recovery. First, let's take a look at what can get in the way.

IDENTIFYING AND
OVERCOMING OBSTACLES

There are many obstacles in the first hours or days of trying to reach recovery. It helps if you're prepared for what may happen. It becomes like walking into a minefield, one misstep and we could hurt ourselves or someone beside us. You may hear or read something in those first moments, which caused you to feel the need to get up and walk out physically or mentally from a plan that is designed to help you. Walking out now can be a disastrous life decision you may later regret.

We like common sense. When Sam Walton started his company Wal-Mart, he used a very simple tool: the multi-lane check out stalls. He saw a problem and figured out how to fix it: people were coming into large box stores but had trouble getting out of them. His solution was adding checkout lanes. A simple change helped create the largest retail store in the world.

We try to take that same logic to recovery. We have to see the problem before we can fix it. This analogy of the big box store can be compared to the recovery industry as a whole. It is easy to get in and hard to get out. Recovery 2-Day™ created a faster checkout lane.

This chapter is to warn you that, as you enter this recovery industry, in many cases, there may not be a safety net underneath you. By using the term "recovery industry" we mean the entire range of services, from courts to inpatient and outpatient rehabilitations, as well as methodology of self-help groups awaiting a person, the client, who enters that industry looking for help. We use the word "treatment" synonymously with recovery industry.

Withdrawal symptoms of most substance problems form a cluster of personal obstacles. Self-motivation is one issue. The, *What's in it for me* thought, if experienced as *nothing or loss only*, creates a personal obstacle. However, if your personal gains outweigh your loss, it creates a feeling of self-improvement, self-commitment, and self-continuance, which is the start of self-development, which makes room for the natural raising of our self-esteem. Distrust moves to trust, if only for a moment.

Another obstacle you need to overcome is magical thinking. This is the idea that someone else will do it for you, that everything will work out and that it will just be okay. This is called "magical thinking."

Your recovery will require you to invest in yourself to get well. First, you must commit to a plan, and then you have to continue with the plan. One of the leading factors in a failed recovery is the idea that once detoxified, you believe that now everything will be okay.

Please realize that detoxification (detox) is not treatment. Detox is only the first stage; detox is a process of getting the substance out of your body in a safe place under medical supervision.

MAGICAL THINKING?

We will describe two extreme examples of widely accepted recovery philosophies: the "have it your way, everything will be okay, magical thinking," approach or the opposite end of the spectrum, the punishment method of recovery, which beats down the person with the phrase, "You're in denial."

Have it your way rarely works. This ambivalence acts like a shoulder shrug, signifying a "whatever." Let us imagine a scenario of a person who enters a hospital with cancer. In an interview in the doctor's office, the doctor and patient discuss which treatment is best. Although the most accepted treatment is radiation and chemotherapy, a bystander says, "Have it your way." The patient shrugs his shoulders and says. "Whatever."

Now, let us consider another example, but this time, you enter a room called Recovery. You are greeted warmly and welcomingly, but then everyone just walks off. They all assume you can figure it out on your own.

Magical thinking or ambivalence leaves you in a dilemma. What will be of value in your recovery process, and what will not? What does it mean when someone says to you, "Take what you want and leave the rest." This is commonly called "Have it your way recovery."

This magical thinking assumes that the newly arriving people, seeking help and answers, will figure it out sooner or later. But the lack of any self-involvement inevitably creates frustration. For a treatment plan to be effective, it must be practical and clear. We don't want you asking for help, and then having to guess on your own what will work and what will not. *You need a plan, showing you what to do, and then you need to do it.* This is why in our preface we asked that you have trust and hope.

However, we are not telling you that you do not have choices. What we're saying is whichever choice you make for a program of recovery, you need to commit to doing it in its entirety, and not pick over its bones to decide the elements that you will do and will not do. For Recovery 2-Day™ to be effective, you need to make a commitment to try all the tools we offer, before you are free to decide which is the most effective for you personally.

So in one corner we have the "Do whatever you want" method of recovery, which obviously does not produce results, since it does nothing and merely hopes for the best by means of magical thinking.

PUNISHMENT THINKING?
Recovery cannot be experienced as punishment.

Another extreme in recovery approaches is the "We need to break you, to make you." Using punishment as an attempt to make you see you have problem, the industry labels this as being in denial. Once a person is determined or labeled as being in denial, then all types of punishment is attempted in order to break it. This is driven by years of industry belief that drug addiction or alcoholism is a moral issue. Again, common sense needs to be used. Since substance dependence is a potential life or freedom threatening problem, we must treat it seriously. When recovery is felt as punishment as we stated earlier, we defeat our purpose of helping.

We need to look at the use of humiliation. Humiliation harms people. Breaking someone for his or her own good, is subjective at best. And if left up to laypeople to determine the breaking or the amount of breaking needed, we see how cruel and unusual punishment can quickly seem normal.

Relax, breathe, exhale: Recovery 2-Day™ is not here to humiliate you, punish you, break you, or label you.

The simple logic of recovery is that if you do not see it as rewarding or gaining something, you will not do it voluntarily. To promote continuance, you have to see a good reason to continue doing something.

In any group, abuse of power can be and often is the reason for many failures. All this model takes is a person in authority over a person who is powerless. If the person with power views their own treatment experience as being victimized, they seek out a person to pay forward the ill treatment they withstood. This creates victimization for the person that follows in their footsteps. And professional jealousy exists as well. What happens, for example, if a layperson becomes the keeper of the professional person for 30 to 90 days? The poor man becomes king for a day. Sometimes, that is attractive to some; it's payback time!

It seems only natural they would inflict their pain onto the next person, entering their reach and perhaps add a few twists for fun. In an effort to make a person feel powerless, power is needed to inflict punishment. But the people being treated this way came here looking for help, not abuse.

We believe that systems that beat people with a you are in denial punishment are detrimental, and it's one reason why so many people who seek help, leave without getting it.

Let us talk about the most painful obstacle, which is being, out of compliance. This means you're under a court-ordered or board supervised, a mandate or sentence and you have not met that sentence.

Let us also be clear about the intent of the courts or medical/professional review boards. Initially they were created to give a person a chance to avoid jails or loss of license. So the process in theory is good. The problem is that if the person or persons sitting in judgment are not aware of the problem in all of its complexity, then it is merely treated as a moral issue, and judgment can be quite harsh. Then recovery systems are merely corrals or holding tanks for the jails. The policing is done by laypeople, which can be frightening if we look closely at the model currently used by both review systems.

Let us take for an example a critical care doctor who drank while under a medical review. This occurred over an eight year period.

This doctor has spent over $250,000 in treatment for being out of compliance. This because the general recovery market for treatment runs in the $1,000 to $50,000+, with the average treatment stay ranging from 30 to 90 days. Obviously, it does not take long to run up a financial mess, not including the aftercare costs of biweekly screening and licensing monitors. This expense is added to the situation created from having the problem in the first place, so difficulties are compounded. Then we have the men and women facing another type of compliance order, a court order, which involves remaining substance free for a set period of time. Prison is the alternative; one must comply and remain substance free. The problem is obvious, the penalty is clear; the medical condition is not addressed. Basically the courts/boards are saying, *Just quit or else.* The "or else" can be expensive and out of most people's reach.

Our doctor friend was sent to treatment to be in compliance, or his medical license would be lost. He was forced to shovel horse manure to promote humility in the hopes of breaking his attitude, making the doctor humble. Since the attitude towards doctors is that they are arrogant and have violated a medical ethos, the approach is to teach them humility. The cost of shoveling the horse manure was $55,000.00 cash. This person entering the horse manure shoveling treatment therapy relapsed on the day of graduation. If shoveling manure is a treatment, than we all need bigger yards and more shovels.

This is not to imply or say that all treatment or treatment facilities are bad or faulty - absolutely NOT.

The fact is that inpatient and outpatient treatments are a highly effective staging area, or entrance, to help millions of people who need help. These people then leave rehab and enter the self-help industry.

Here are the places people go for help:

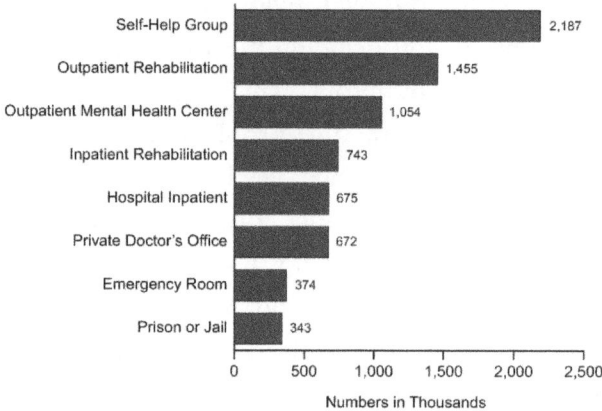

Self-Help Group	2,187
Outpatient Rehabilitation	1,455
Outpatient Mental Health Center	1,054
Inpatient Rehabilitation	743
Hospital Inpatient	675
Private Doctor's Office	672
Emergency Room	374
Prison or Jail	343

Numbers in Thousands

Results from the 2008 NSDUH: National Findings, SAMHSA, OAS

Our doctor was actually lucky, in one sense. He could afford inpatient rehabilitation. He simply paid a lot of money, in our opinion, to shovel horse manure.

If we examine this $55,000 treatment, the doctor complied with a board, and he shoveled horse manure. The doctor graduated and the doctor drank. Upon graduation, he was told, as the final instruction, to attend meetings.

What happens after treatment from inpatient or outpatient rehabilitation? Was it necessary or helpful for the doctor to be treated with daily humiliation in the hope of breaking him? Did he spend $55,000 just to be told, *Go to meetings?*

Imagine a person with a disease such as lung cancer or diabetes. Now, transfer the treatment the doctor was prescribed, daily manure shoveling, to the lung cancer patient, or to the diabetic, and you understand why we say using humiliation as a cure does not work, and needs to be discontinued.

Always comply with your board or court order, no matter if you feel you are innocent or guilty, no matter if you feel justified. No matter what, comply. We are sorry you are caught in this punishment system, especially if you find yourself shoveling manure as a treatment plan. An apology here will not make your problems go away. But after it's over, choose to follow our treatment plan to truly get well, and we can help you avoid the certain consequences of falling back into being "out of compliance."

RECOVERY STRESS LIST

We coined a term, Recovery Stress. The stressors that you face now and in the immediate future when you begin the recovery process are identifiable. Part of a healthy short-term plan in your recovery is to address what is happening in your life currently. You'll need to inspect your landscape, including who is in your life now. Then you need to imagine what that same landscape may look like without a substance problem. Common sense tells you that some things, not all things, but some things will change. It's important to be aware of the dangers changes may present to you. As you prepare for a future without a substance problem, identify what may change will help the transition. Possible changes include feeling like a fish out of water, or having a sense of lost identity, of simply the strangeness of having the substance problem removed.

If you can anticipate where stress comes from, then you can assess how much attention you have to pay to it. This simple list, called the Recovery Stress List, will help in this process.

Take out a piece of paper and pen. On the top of the paper, make a list of people who are in your life currently. Who is awaiting your return? Whether you are creating this in a rehab, treatment center, or home, it does not matter. You need this information to help you identify potential stressors. List all the people in your life 2-Day. This information is the entrance to discovery of where your stress or potential stress will come from.

Q1: Who is in your life currently? In addition, consider under what conditions do you use a substance? At home, work, socially, drug house?

Where do you live? Who do you live with? How often will you be in contact with the people on the list?

Now there are two judgment questions that we need to address honestly:

Do they (the person on the list), have a substance problem?

Do they (the person on the list) support, play a role in, or have an influence in your recovery?

You need this list to determine who you can anticipate recovery stress from and what actions or plans you can develop to address the feelings of stress before they take over.

Recovery Stress List example:

Q1: Who is in my life 2-Day?
• My parents and family members Name of spouse, partner, boyfriend, girlfriend etc...
• My spouse's/partner's/boyfriend's/girlfriend's parents
• My drug dealer's name (a common question by many Do I list this? Yes)
• My drug places (where we spend a lot of time, finding, selling, buying, etc...)
• My drinking friends (bars, etc...)
• My weekly pattern (do I go out each Friday night and do what?)
• My employers (names of them, be specific, not vague)
• My coworkers(names of them, be specific, not vague)
• My kids (if present, living with us or not)
• My close friends (yes, name names since each one will need to be examined)

Once you have that part completed, look at each person you have listed and ask **Q2:** Do they have a substance problem?

Q2: Do they have a substance problem?	Yes / No and Maybe/ Not Sure
My parents and family members	Yes, mother drinks, yes father drinks
Name of spouse/partner/boyfriend/ girlfriend/etc…	No
My spouse's, partner's, boyfriend's, girlfriend's parents and family members	Yes, they take drugs
My drug dealer's name (a common question by many, Do I list this? Yes)	This is a place to avoid, applying common sense
My drug places (where we spend a lot of time, finding, selling, buying, etc…)	This is a place to avoid, applying common sense
My drinking friends (bars, etc…)	Some are problems some are not
My weekly pattern (do I go out each Friday night and do what?)	Favorite bar was X
My employers (names of them, be specific, not vague)	Seems safe
My coworkers(names of them, be specific, not vague)	Some use, some don't
My kids (if present, living with us or not)	No
My close friends (yes, name names since each one will need to be examined)	Some do, so do not

Common sense tells you that not all people on your list can or will be avoided. What happens, for example, if your parents use drugs or drink and you are underage and living at home? If you know your co-workers enjoy a drink now and then, how do you prepare for questions like, Would you like to join us this Friday night? Or what do you say when you return to work after being in rehab and you are asked, "Where have you been?"

Q3: Do they support my recovery?	Yes / No and Maybe/ Not Sure
My parents and family members	Yes, but they will continue to drink
Name of spouse, partner, boyfriend, girlfriend etc…	Not sure
My spouse's, partner's, boyfriend's, girlfriend's parents and family members	Yes
My drug dealer's name (a common question by many Do I list this? Yes)	They will call me and want me back
My drug places (where we spend a lot of time, finding, selling, buying, etc…)	NO
My drinking friends (bars, etc…)	Some will, some won't and some won't care
My weekly pattern (do I go out each Friday night and do what?)	Assess future plans
My employers (names of them, be specific, not vague)	Seems safe
My coworkers(names of them, be specific, not vague)	Some will, some won't some won't care
My kids (if present, living with us or not)	Yes,
My close friends (yes, name names since each one will need to be examined)	Some do, so do not

The Recovery Stress List will show you that during your short-term recovery you will feel stress. Not all of it can be avoided but it can be mitigated by being prepared.

BUILDING ANOTHER HALLWAY
IN RECOVERY 2-DAY™

What do you feel when you see someone slip, lapse, and reenter full-blown relapse? Do you think that this is purely a lack of willingness, and the person who did not try hard enough or simply did not want to quit? Or are you aware that many people are forced into a recovery that they were never going to accept in the first place. The fact is that of the 20.8 million who need or are seen as having a problem, 25% or 5 million, do not want to quit. First, if a person does not want to quit, it should not be viewed as *relapse or failure of treatment*. Even if they attended substance treatment or face consequences of any sort, since they did not accept there was a strong enough reason to remain substance free, including personal loss of freedom or social rejection.

This means that 15 million people *do* want to quit and they can be helped. The biggest obstacle and most misunderstood obstacle to remaining permanently substance free is relapse.

Relapse is a horrible thing to witness or experience. Watching a person walk away from being well is a stomach-turning event. It is especially terrible when this person is part of a group of men and women that most recovery self-help groups discount: they are afflicted by a mental illness that is masked by a substance abuse or dependence problem.

Did the person who slipped, lapsed, or entered full relapse ever really want to quit, was quitting too hard, or was there another reason? The United States Veterans Affairs defines alcoholism and drug addiction as willful misconduct. It is seen as a self-inflicted wound.

This makes it sound as if it is entirely the individual's choice to get well or not, and it discounts the disease concept of substance abuse or dependence.

Of the same 20.8 million people with a substance abuse or dependence problem, 10% have Severe Mental Illness (SMI) and of that 2.5 million, only 11% receive treatment. This means we are NOT helping those with SMI, and yes, clinical depression is considered as SMI. What do we tell 10% of the people who enter recovery looking for help with a substance problem but who used a substance to mask or treat their mental illness?

The only answer must be for these people to *seek professional help*. If they need help with their substance problem after they have treated their SMI, then and only then would recovery be a part of the long-term solution. Until the mental disorder is treated, we will never meet or treat the real person or underlying problems.

However, the problem becomes the person with SMI, and it must be separated from substance abuse or dependence to reveal the hidden truth, and finding that takes time. This also reveals the absolute value of treatment in medically supervised rehabs, which under the proper medical diagnosis moves recovery in the right areas. This means that 10% of the people looking for recovery are finding they have much deeper issues than simply a substance problem. This also explains why longer-term in-patient treatment is recommended, since a trained medical staff would have more time to discover and address problems other than a substance problem. Even so, cost is always a factor. Who can afford to be away from work or family for three, six, or twelve months? This keeps the self-help groups in the treatment industry, since they are the cheapest after care available, but they are not always going to be the most effective for all people who seek help. This also explains the explosion we see in the recovery/treatment industry, ranging typically from religious to secular solutions. Rarely, however, do the treatments combine all three in a holistic way, and offer medical, religious, and secular solutions.

The question of "Do you think you have a problem" has to shift now. Has detox revealed more than a substance problem? Sometimes you may find that you have parallel problems that must have parallel treatments As laypersons, we are not qualified to do this.

Who knows and how do we access the mental stability of a person looking for help? We cannot, since we are not medical professionals or doctors. We must however acknowledge that it is a possibility.

Perhaps in the future we can develop a better working relationship, alliances with the medical professionals that treat SMI to the point of having them attend self-help group meetings or at least build a network with the medical professionals to refer our visitors to the right places for help. Yes, this would mean inviting the therapists and psychotherapists and psychiatrists to the self-help group industry. This we believe was the initial intent of the after care industry of treatment centers or rehabs that have become the entrance into most recovery systems. The problem, of course, is funding. Who pays the salaries of the professionals since treatment or rehab costs tens of thousands of dollars? This is the reason the self-help group is so widely popular. It is the cheap treatment, but is it effective for the 10% who need long-term medical professional help? And yes is the answer, if and only if the self-help groups acknowledge the need for outside medical and medicinal professional help.

This means the question we asked, "Do you want to get well," comes with a disclaimer of sorts: Will you seek professional help if you need it to accomplish this, as part of your continued self-help treatment? *Common sense tells us that only treating one of the problems instead of addressing all other problems never addresses the entire problem.*

This tells us that 10% or 2.5 million people with a substance problem and other mental illness should be seeking multiple paths to mental health, which means we must start merging or forming alliances. The hallway of Recovery 2-Day™ promotes a healthy return to do this. We will attempt to join another 2. Our name 2-Day constantly shifts to being more inclusive, and we must see and accept the medical professional as an integral part of most long-term treatment for 2-Day's clients. For any recovery system to be helpful, 2.5 million men and women require more than a self-help group can offer, to achieve mental health and life without a substance problem. The industry must adapt to accepting the fact that we cannot solve all the problems a person brings when they seek help, since for many it takes months to determine what if any other problems exist?

We must drop the idea that we can solve all our problems, or that we have all the answers. We cannot. However, not all is lost. Recovery 2-Day™ builds the hallway to enter the right treatment once the problem is properly and medically diagnosed. There should be no shame or guilt associated with seeking professional help in your search for getting well.

BRAIN DISEASE 101

We need to first define the words: disease and mental disorder. Since now we are getting personal, did you just think we called you a name? By using the word brain disease did that make you sit back in your chair and pause, with a feeling of "not me."

There is a broad definition of disease and a narrow definition. The broad definition is this: Diseases are what people go to doctors for, they presumably do so because they believe doctors can help them (whether this is true or not.)

The narrow definition of disease holds that every disease has an underlying biochemical, physiological, or anatomical abnormality, the nature of which may not be known.

Clinical Textbook of Addictive Disorder: Richard J. Frances M.D., Sheldon I Miller M.D.

Mental disorder: Whatever its original cause, it must currently be considered a manifestation of a behavioral, psychological, or biological dysfunction in the individual.

Source: American Psychiatric Association Diagnostic Statistical Manual of Mental Disorders Forth edition Text Revision. Washington, DC, American Psychiatric Association, 2000.

Educating the public and the men and women working in the industry is a daunting task. Many doctors continue to believe dependence is merely a behavioral problem.

> *Dr. Raoul Walsh in an article published in the November 1995 issue of Lancet supports the contention that physicians have negative views about alcoholics. He cites empirical data showing physicians continue to have stereotypical attitudes about alcoholics and that non-psychiatrists tend to view alcohol problems as principally the concern of psychiatrists. He also contends that many doctors have negative attitudes towards patients with alcohol problems because the bulk of their clinical exposure is with late-stage alcohol dependence.*
>
> *Based on my experiences working in the addiction field for the past 10 years, I believe many, if not most, health professionals still view alcohol addiction as a willpower or conduct problem and are resistant to look at it as a disease. Part of the problem is that medical schools provide little time to study alcoholism or addiction and post-graduate training usually deals only with the end result of addiction or alcohol/drug-related diseases.*

Source: Managing alcoholism as a disease Thomas R. Hobbs, Ph.D., M.D., was the medical director of the Physicians' Health Programs (PHP). The PHP, a program of The Educational and Scientific Trust of the Pennsylvania Medical Society, is a confidential advocacy service for physicians suffering from impairing conditions.

Substance abuse or misuse would be a better description, of a brain disorder while substance dependence, which is a complex brain disease is typically only taught in treatment facilities, and understood by science professionals, but is not taught or offered in most self-help recovery groups. Many years of medical progress have been missing since the first attempts were made to address the issue. Self-help groups are the largest treatment group in the recovery industry.

Self-Help Group	2,187
Outpatient Rehabilitation	1,455
Outpatient Mental Health Center	1,054
Inpatient Rehabilitation	743
Hospital Inpatient	675
Private Doctor's Office	672
Emergency Room	374
Prison or Jail	343

Numbers in Thousands

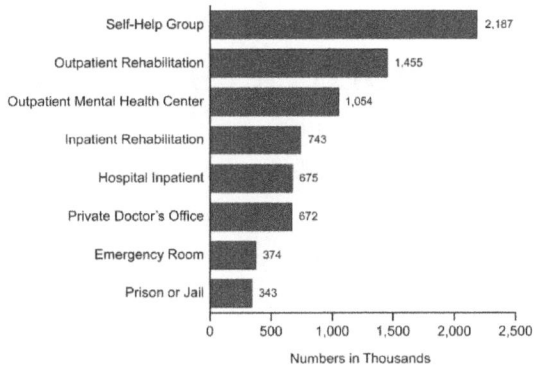

Results from the 2008 NSDUH: National Findings, SAMHSA, OAS

We need to understand that the brain controls our entire body. What does that mean to someone suffering with substance problems? Affect the brain and you affect the entire body. Damage the brain, and we damage the owner of it. Most people still believe it is a moral issue, since they view addiction as a self-inflicted problem, willful misconduct, never understanding it is a chemically induced change in the brain neurotransmitters pathway that creates the involuntary chemical dependency dysregulation. We also need to accept that different drugs affect different parts of the brain, making the slogan a drug is a drug is a drug a false statement. If that were medically true, then the heart patient could take alcohol or crack to cure their arrhythmia instead nitroglycerin. Certain slogans must be discarded with logic and facts. Many treatments appear similar, but the damage is different. This allows for different treatments, as the damage is revealed over a time period.

Substance problems move from choice to compulsion. Compulsion means a force that makes someone do something, even if it is harmful."I drank against my own will" or "I drugged against my own will" are common statements made by those men and women that entered dependence. Dependence became an involuntary action.

HOW DOES ADDICTION
TAKE HOLD IN THE BRAIN?

The rewarding effects of drugs of abuse come from large and rapid upsurges in dopamine, a neurochemical critical to stimulating feelings of pleasure and to motivating behavior. The rapid dopamine rush from drugs of abuse mimics but greatly exceeds in intensity and duration the feelings that occur in response to such pleasurable stimuli as the sight or smell of food, for example. Repeated exposure to large, drug-induced dopamine surges has the insidious consequence of ultimately blunting the response of the dopamine system to everyday stimuli. Thus, the drug disturbs a person's normal hierarchy of needs and desires and substitutes new priorities concerned with procuring and using the drug.

Drug abuse also disrupts the brain circuits involved in memory and control over behavior. Memories of the drug experience can trigger craving in people exposed to stressful situations or to people, places, or things they associate with their former drug use. Control over behavior becomes compromised because the affected frontal brain regions are what a person needs to exert inhibitory control over desires and emotions.

That is why addiction is a brain disease. As a person's reward circuitry becomes increasingly dulled and desensitized by drugs, nothing else can compete with them—food, family, and friends lose their relative value, while the ability to curb the need to seek and use drugs evaporates. Ironically and cruelly, eventually even the drug loses its ability to reward, but the compromised brain leads addicted people to pursue it, anyway; the memory of the drug has become more powerful than the drug itself.

Source: Nora Volkow, M.D., Director, National Institute on Drug Abuse

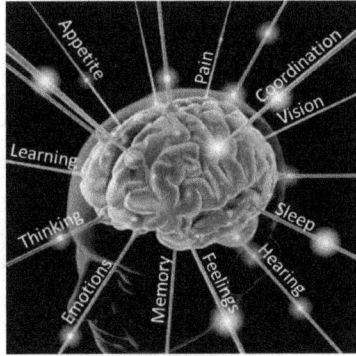

IMAGE 1

Carlton Erickson, Ph.D, in his book *"The Science of Addiction"* describes neurotransmitter dysregulation and that different chemicals, drugs affect different areas of neurotransmitter sites in the brain.

If you look at Image 1 above, you'll see simultaneous responsibilities of the brain. Different areas of our brain control different functions, such as our decision-making abilities or memory, and more importantly the rewards/pleasure part of our brains. Some brain functions are involuntary such as heartbeat or eyes blinking. Voluntary brain action, choice, creates individuals, some that prefer red meat to poultry. Where choice comes into play in abuse and dependence is where most people never pay attention. Choice is lost once an involuntary chemical dependence in the brain is reached, turning from choice to irrational compulsion also known as brain disease, the loss of thought and reason of our cognitive thought process. This is why so many believe it is self-inflicted, since it started in most cases voluntarily. Typically what is true is the chase – the sense of euphoria the drug delivers, not the disease. And not everyone who takes a drug becomes dependent. However, anyone can misuse a substance, not everyone that misuses or abused a substance, becomes dependent. Each individual has entirely different brain transmitter sites since we are unique genetically.

The reason this concept is important to understand is our brain delegates information and instructions to its different areas. What happens to the brain when we introduce drugs and alcohol to it? The influence on our brains affects over different time periods, our entire body, in increased amounts (tolerance). We do create damage, some irreversible in different areas. What would happen if we damage our emotional part of our brain? What happens if we damage our memory parts of our brain or sensory, speech, balance and movement? A person can damage the vision part of the brain and still hear, but would never see again. How these events, or emotions-memories, are stored and under what conditions they were encoded, are significant in how we see the world.

We need to understand how these chemicals, drugs or alcohol, act on our brains. They mimic or trick the brain. Since our brains are compartmentalized in function but work in parallel to each other, different areas are affected. Most drugs and alcohol affect the reward/pleasure zone of our brains, the Limbic System that regulates our emotions (anger, fear, love) and memory. All parts connect to our cognitive thought processes. A different section of our brain (your forehead area) is called the Orbital-Frontal Cortex (OFC), where thinking, reasoning, and decisions are made, typically based on emotional-memory or feelings. Memory is stored as sensory, like the passing smell of a cup of hot chocolate, or the scent of flowers. Short-term memory moves the sensory memory to a staging area, like our ability to sing along with a song. Long-term memory moved the short-term memory to a reusable memory; and we attach feeling to the memory like I love that song. Another example of long-term memory is remembering multiplication tables or riding a bike by repetition. The OFC does not fully develop until a person reaches the age of twenty-five or twenty-six years of age.

Notice the words cognitive thought processes. This is where most of the research and progress of substance problems is being researched. A general term for psychotherapy called Cognitive Behavioral Therapy (CBT) is now the preferred method for treatment therapists and medical professionals. CBT uses terms such as coping skills and self-awareness, by teaching behavior skills through educating the client and requires a good - safe relationship with the therapist. Aaron Beck, M.D developed Cognitive Therapy (CT) in 1960 as an effective therapy for men and women that suffered from depression. David Burns author of *Feeling Good* made CBT popular in the 80's. *Source: National Association of Cognitive-Behavioral Therapists*

Logic tells us that if we damaged the brain, we must treat the brain. Treat the brain and we treat the body. This logic is fairly easy to see, if a heart condition were diagnosed, we would not treat the toenail to solve it. We would treat the heart condition. The same is true of a brain disorder or disease: we treat the affected area. We will not have time to address diet, but that too is important since many have such poor dietary habits. We are saying that personal health needs an active participant. Osmosis, rather than deliberate learning, will not work.

Hope is needed to move a person from simple acknowledgement to actively believing in his or her ability to overcome the initial problem. The first problem is removing the toxins from our bodies, a medical detoxification (detox) is highly recommended. It is not advisable to detox without medical assistance due to the certain health issues that can happen while our bodies adapt to sudden chemical changes in our brains. Seizure, depression and heart failures are common withdrawal symptoms, as well as suicides

In 2003, there were 348,830 nonfatal emergency department (ED) visits by adults aged 18 or older who had harmed themselves. Research suggests that there may be between 8 and 25 attempted

suicides for every suicide death. As with suicide completions, risk factors for attempted suicide in adults include depression and substance use.

Results from the 2008 NSDUH: National Findings, SAMHSA, OAS

Once detoxed, we must have cognitive tools to inspect and properly interpret the problem.

Then we have to develop more cognitive skills to take on the life problems that follow. This allows a person to reroute the damaged emotional-memory with new experiences, by acquiring knowledge and undamaged emotional-memories. This tells us that our treatment plan needs to have tools, coping skills, which help us develop as we change. Our old negative long-term memories must be rerouted by new positive, short-term and long-term memory. They must adapt to our needs as we change, moving from the abnormal physical state of not using to the new normal state of life without a substance. In short, our behaviors must change.

DO YOU THINK
YOU HAVE A PROBLEM?

Now, we will see who is doing what? It helps to see that you are not the only one that has this substance problem; in fact, a large part of our population does.

A recent study from the Department of Health shows from age 12 up below in Image 2.

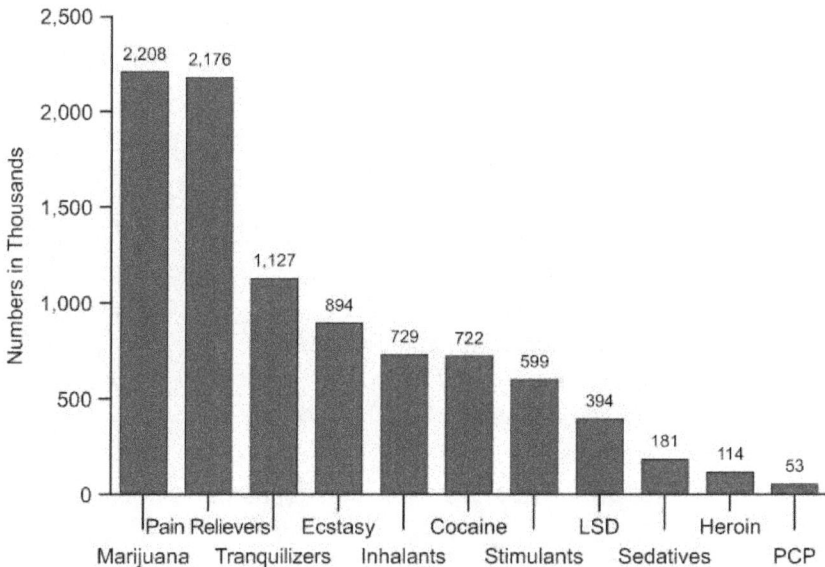

IMAGE 2

- *The OAS Report is published periodically by the Office of Applied Studies, Substance Abuse and Mental Health Services Administration (SAMHSA)*

- *Alcohol studies from the same source show More than one fifth (23.3 percent) of persons aged 12 or older participated in binge drinking at least once in the 30 days prior to the survey in 2007. This translates to about 57.8 million people. The rate in 2007 is similar to the rate in 2006 (23.0 percent).*

- *Slightly more than half of Americans aged 12 or older reported being current drinkers of alcohol in the 2008 survey (51.6 percent). This translates to an estimated 129.0 million people, which is similar to the 2007 estimate of 126.8 million people (51.1 percent).*

- *More than one fifth (23.3 percent) of persons aged 12 or older participated in binge drinking at least once in the 30 days prior to the survey in 2008. This translates to about 58.1 million people. The rate in 2008 is the same as the rate in 2007 (23.3 percent).*

- *In 2008, heavy drinking was reported by 6.9 percent of the population aged 12 or older, or 17.3 million people. This percentage is the same as the rate of heavy drinking in 2007 (6.9 percent).*

Facts are helpful when we look at substance problems at this confusing time of our lives. There are many opinions and urban legends that must be addressed. Most of the progress made in treatment and research has remained outside the reach of those that need it for various reasons.

We come to the most important questions. *Do I think I have a problem,* and if so *what happens next?* Facts need to replace opinion and theory, so we can attempt to avoid another debate. That is exactly what we here at Recovery 2-Day™ will do. We will show the medical criterion of Substance Abuse and Substance Dependence.

We must be clear in what defines substance abuse and what defines substance dependence. Then, each person can look at the definitions and honestly make an assessment.

Once that hurdle is faced honestly, a person can rethink the internal question, *Do I think I have a problem?*

After the external medical definition is examined and internalized, then, that same person may ask, *What can I do about it?*

Coming to that conclusion is never easy, since it involves considering being separated from a substance that you became dependent upon and the idea of living without it (a long-term treatment plan). Blame is an obstacle for many people. You may still hold onto the idea that it's someone else's fault. To help remove obstacles, we recommend you begin with this simple tool:

It is a simple list, generated by a question or series of questions. In Recovery 2-Day™ we call these lists tools, and we introduce them as soon as you arrive. You will need a notebook of paper and a pen. The next tool is one of many we will show you how to use.

The Regrets List

- Do you have any regrets regarding your use of alcohol or drugs?
- Have you perhaps lost someone or something? What has brought you to this time in your life, now sitting here reading a book that deals with substance abuse and substance dependence?
- Stop here for a moment and reflect on your life up to this moment 2-Day.
- Ask yourself Do I have any regrets with using drugs or drinking?
- *Keep this list, and we will use it later in another tool.*

Now, take a piece of paper and pen. Avoid the temptation to do this in your mind, since your mind will often minimize the past events with It's or I'm, not that bad. Often you may be surprised when you see things written in your own hand. *For clarity's sake, when we say take out some paper and pen, we need you to go and grab some paper and a pen. It will only take a moment to do this.*

On the top of the paper simply write, "I regret" or "My regrets list."

Now simply be honest. No one is going to see this list.

HERE IS AN EXAMPLE
OF A SIMPLE LIST
I REGRET...

Quitting school

Getting kicked out of college

Fighting with my parents/friends

Cheating on my spouse/partner

Lying at home

Getting fired

Using drugs

Wrecking the car

Losing my family

Living on the streets

Relapsing

Becoming what I became

Missing my parent's funeral

Losing my children

Using drugs in front of my children

Losing my parents' respect

Losing my life's savings

Etc...

Losing my license (any type)

Leaving home

Hitting my spouse/partner

Lying at work

Getting caught

I didn't want this to happen

Going to jail/prison

Embarrassing myself

Using people

Losing a career

Going to 10 treatment centers

Cussing out my friends

Missing my children's birthdays

Selling myself

Using drugs with my children

Losing myself respect

Stealing

The Regrets List is very insightful and can be long or short, depending on how long a person lived with the results the consequences of years of substance abuse or dependence. We also know the risk of supplying an example. Do not use this example as a check list. Write your own regrets list. This is merely an example of a regrets list.

Our lists allow us to consider whether these events would have happened had drinking or taking drugs not been involved.

WHAT IS SUBSTANCE ABUSE?

Now, with your regrets list in hand and fresh in your mind, take a look at the medical criteria and see if you land in the criteria of abuse established by the American Psychiatric Association Diagnostic Statistical Manual of Mental Disorders Forth edition Text Revision. Washington, DC, American Psychiatric Association, 2000.

DSM-IV-TR Substance Abuse Criteria

A: Substance abuse is defined as a maladaptive pattern of substance use leading to clinically significant impairment or distress as manifested by one (or more) of the following, occurring within a 12-month period:

Recurrent substance use resulting in a failure to fulfill major role obligations at work, school, or home (e.g. such as repeated absences or poor work performance related to substance use; substance-related absences, suspensions, or expulsions from school; or neglect of children or household).

Recurrent substance use in situations in which it is physically hazardous (such as driving an automobile or operating a machine when impaired by substance use).

Recurrent substance-related legal problems (such as arrests for substance related disorderly conduct).

Continued substance use despite having persistent or recurrent social or interpersonal problems caused or exacerbated by the effects of the substance (for example, arguments with spouse about consequences of intoxication and physical fights).

B: The symptoms for abuse have never met the criteria for dependence for this class of substance.

Obviously, this criterion of involving abuse misuse is very broad and grim and depressing. Some of the people in this category can, with very little assistance quit, or moderate. More importantly, we at Recovery 2-Day™ do not look down on amounts taken. If a person believes there is a problem, the amount taken is not our concern. There is no competition regarding who, drank or drugged more or who drank or drugged less. That type of negative pride has no value here. Now, let us take our regrets list and compare it to the medical criteria of dependence, established by the American Psychiatric Association Diagnostic Statistical Manual of Mental Disorders.

WHAT IS SUBSTANCE DEPENDENCE?

DSM-IV-TR *Substance Dependence Criteria*

Substance dependence is defined as a maladaptive pattern of substance use leading to clinically significant impairment or distress, as manifested by <u>three (or more)</u> of the following, occurring any time in the same 12-month period:

<u>Tolerance</u>, as defined by either of the following:

A need for markedly increased amounts of the substance to achieve intoxication or the desired effect.

Markedly diminished effect with continued use of the same amount of the substance.

<u>Withdrawal</u>, as manifested by either of the following:

The characteristic withdrawal syndrome for the substance (refer to Criteria A and B of the criteria sets for Withdrawals from the specific substances)

The same (or closely related) substance is taken to relieve or avoid withdrawal symptoms.

The substance is often taken in larger amounts or over a longer period than intended.

> *There is a persistent desire or unsuccessful efforts to cut down or control substance use.*
>
> *A great deal of time is spent in activities necessary to obtain the substance, use the substance, or recover from its effects.*
>
> *Important social, occupational, or recreational activities are given up or reduced because of substance use.*
>
> *The substance use is continued despite knowledge of having a persistent physical or psychological problem that is likely to have been caused or exacerbated by the substance (for example, current cocaine use despite recognition of cocaine-induced depression or continued drinking despite recognition that an ulcer was made worse by alcohol consumption).*

When comparing your regrets list to the medical criteria, were past or current substance use, misuse, or dependence mentioned? Facts allow us to determine if we fall in one or the other criteria, not both. Clearly now, we begin to see, there no need or value in being labeled. We must be properly diagnosed, so we can make informed decisions about solving the problem.

Do you understand the logic of removing the obstacle of labeling with this simple question: "Do you, the reader, believe you have a problem?" With this ever-so-simple question, we avoid being distracted and sidelined in discussions, war stories that describe amounts consumed, or levels of progression from substance abuse to dependence. If you believe you have a problem, we can move on. If you are not sure, we can move on. If you do not believe you have a problem, we can move on.

Since it is not our job to try to convince anyone there is a problem, we have focused on finding a method to solve the problem, simply because we agree a problem exists. If you agree with our methods, then you will shift from being here reluctantly to voluntarily. You volunteer and do what we have done to get well. Abstinence is the long-term goal of a good treatment plan.

The beauty of this method also removes the need to self-label, just like the term substance abuse or substance dependence removes the need to identify the substance. If you have a crack dependence problem, or an alcohol dependence problem, or an opiate dependence problem, the substance becomes less important. Medically, the problem is simply defined as substance abuse or dependence. It is not important to any of us here at Recovery 2-Day™ if the substance you were dependent on was a street drug, a bottle of vodka, or a bottle of pain pills. It can, however, determine how long it may take you to get well, since different chemicals affect the brain differently. Some men and women have done severe damage to their brain and body and physically need longer to heal and restore their health. This should not mean they delay getting well, which begins the moment they seek help.

Here, we are addressing those who have moved from choice, social use, into abuse, and then into compulsive dependence. For your success, we make the assumption that anyone taking on this issue personally is not here to moderate or return to normal drug use or normal alcohol activities. The people we are addressing are looking for answers and valid tools to solve their problem with substance abuse or dependence. Again, this is more important to us here at Recovery 2-Day™ than labels or self-descriptors.

The regrets list you just produced generates natural questions. What, if anything, did your regrets list reveal? Do you have a problem? Do you want to do anything about it? How can you quit?

We return to our favorite question, our lead-off question, Do _you_ think you have a problem? The emphasis is on you, the reader, who is asking this question. External pressure has perhaps forced you into answering in different ways at different times, but you must try to answer it seriously and as honestly as possible. We are not trying to convert you into anything. The solution to the problem is more important than what brings you here.

If you believe you have a problem, this brings us to the next question:

Do you want to do anything about it? Here, No is a valid response. But is the reason behind the No based solely on external factors? Keeping your job, saving your family or avoiding jail/prison sentences are valid objectives. However, does resolving these external problems fully address the problem you may have developed with either substance abuse or dependence? *No, really I just want to keep my job. My spouse kicked me out and I just want to get back in my home. I'm just here to satisfy the judge or probation/parole officer.* These are common issues heard from many arriving into the recovery industry. Twenty-five percent of men and women are not ready to stop using.

If you have decided you have a problem and you want to do something about it, what are other obstacles in your path? Cost is a factor for everyone. In fact, cost of treatment is the number one reason 7 out of 20 million men and women who seek help never receive help. Moreover, because of costs, this also explains why so many visit self-help groups, called meetings or fellowships. However if the recovery industry is only producing 5% or 10% success, then we have a 90% to 95% failure rate. Recovery 2-Day™'s goal is to bring a measurable and marked improvement to these current statistics.

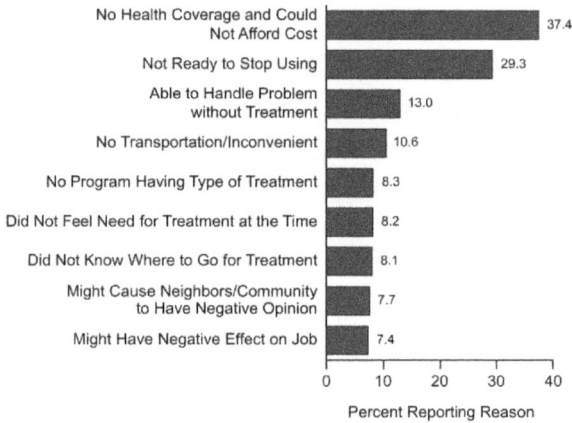

No Health Coverage and Could Not Afford Cost — 37.4
Not Ready to Stop Using — 29.3
Able to Handle Problem without Treatment — 13.0
No Transportation/Inconvenient — 10.6
No Program Having Type of Treatment — 8.3
Did Not Feel Need for Treatment at the Time — 8.2
Did Not Know Where to Go for Treatment — 8.1
Might Cause Neighbors/Community to Have Negative Opinion — 7.7
Might Have Negative Effect on Job — 7.4

Percent Reporting Reason

IMAGE 3

20.8 Million Needing But Not Receiving Treatment for Illicit Drug or Alcohol Use
Results from the 2008 NSDUH: National Findings, SAMHSA, OAS

By looking at the Department of Health statistics for 2008, Image 3, we see the largest group of men and women seeking help find it too expensive. They could not afford to get well.

Do you want to get well?

We have shown you the medical community's position only to show current criteria used in the recovery industry to diagnose substance abuse or substance dependence. That does not mean we are saying, You are one, since only the person asking the question of him or herself can determine this.

Again, to answer a question properly, you need to have the terms defined. You have to know what the criterion is to help answer the question, *Do I want to get well?*

We also know that placing our belief in the medical description of substance problems will immediately cause some to disagree. Having this medical certainty immediately creates denial in those who want to debate it. Some will always insist it is merely a moral issue. Recovery 2-Day™ will point to statements made by the American Medical Association (AMA) and American Psychiatric Association (APA). Both have clearly have ruled on this issue.

This is the **AMA policy**:

H-95.983 Drug Dependencies as Diseases
1.   Endorses the proposition that drug dependencies, including alcoholism, are diseases and that their treatment is a legitimate part of medical practice, and
2.   Encourages physicians, other health professionals, medical and other health related organizations, and government and other policymakers to become more well informed about drug dependencies, and to base their policies and activities on the recognition that drug dependencies are, in fact, diseases. (Res. 113, A-87)
http://www.amaassn.org/ama1/pub/upload/mm/388/alcoholism_treatable.pdf

This is where education becomes invaluable. Once you become educated about the disease, you are ready to self-evaluate. Everything weighs on the outcome of your self-evaluation. It is complicated since we are dealing with unique individuals with unique personalities, culture and environments. Each person arrives in his or her own self-truth differently. Also complicating things is the moving target. As you progress in substance use, the substance may change. Some may have had early signs of a problem with a substance, so they switch to other substances or vice versa. Moreover, everyone involved is frustrated by the unseen damage physically and psychologically a person has sustained. Determining how much damage has been done to a person's brain, chemically altered from years of exposure to a substance, takes time. This damage can only be assessed after the person is successfully detoxed from the substance or substances used. Even then, the full extent of the damage cannot be determined until one or two years of complete abstinence have been achieved.

We know how frightening this feels. Suddenly to find a truth you have been trying to evade is agonizing. Brought on by multiple reasons, ranging from health issues to family problems, legal or employment consequences, or self destructive actions, the illusion or delusion that you don't have a problem finally collapses, and you can admit the truth, if only for an instant. Getting caught could be and often is the first time that this question is faced. Sadly, for many, avoiding getting caught again or evading punishment becomes the challenge, instead of facing the problem.

Equally confusing at this moment of self-admission is the internal upheaval of pain and raw emotion. The distortion in our minds meets itself like the shattering of a mirror. It is as if we have fallen to pieces and, shattered, now face the irrational fear of never being able to be put back together. Utter loss, defeat, and depression are common effects following the admission. This reality is the darkest moment, and if followed up with no help, or no one to guide us, it feels impossible to ever pick ourselves up again.

We normally fly under the flag of, *You don't or won't understand,* and we are convinced that no one could possibly understand how devastating this moment of self-admission feels. Feeling this hopelessness, the common reaction is, *Why bother, I'm hopeless.* While this feels true, feelings are not facts. We also have to fight through the prejudice of terms like mental disorders or mental illness. In our defensiveness we hear, you're crazy, you're insane, which we do not believe. Mental Disorders can be and are treated with success 2-Day. **We can and do get well.** Anyone who has experienced this moment of self-admission understands how difficult it is. The image we see of ourselves in that moment is not to our liking, and we feel that something needs to be done. Something has to change. The sense of loss is immense, and this forces a new insight upon us. *How can I get better?* Our survival instinct reaches for help.

Nevertheless, emotional and feeling states of mind do not help answer the question, *How can I get better?* if we are still battling the question, *Do I have a problem?* This is where the possibility that you are in denial will be the tool used in the recovery industry to break the cycle of *I shouldn't be here, I'm not that bad, I can quit anytime I want.* We are tempted to go back in time, to a place in our memory when drug or alcohol use was not experienced as a problem, called euphoric recall. But in those memories, we were not faced with problems such as losing our jobs, our families, or our freedom. The solution stored in memory, when no external problems existed, defines the solution of how to handle our current problems. Going back in time, however, is not possible. Most of us spend years in euphoric recall, romancing the good old days and pretending they will return. Why can't I just go back to the way it was? For some it take decades to accept the depth of their problem.

While no one likes to feel guilt and shame, the benefit of these emotions and feelings is that they bring these questions to the surface. The moment of self-realization and self-defeat does not last long. Emotions and feelings are transient. Our minds, too, can quickly adapt. The idea of living without the substance is not a pleasant one, our memory, emotions and feelings will search out a new belief, trying to protect its old memory from changing. The new belief can be deceptive, *I'm innocent, I'm not that bad, I shouldn't be here, I am the victim here, and I only had one.* This list of excuses can be as long as our memories allow, avoiding the self-inspection, Do I think I have a problem.

In addition, removing the substance reveals other problems in some. Other mental illnesses may be present, such as, bi-polar, schizophrenia, depression, psychotic, etc. This would create the need for parallel treatment plans, which would treat multiple conditions that would incorporate mental health professionals.

For some, substance use masked or coexisted with other serious mental or physical conditions. Those who need professional assistance must have the freedom to seek that assistance without the judgment that they are less worthy than those who need no such additional help. In fact, many with untreated mental illness have self-medicated for decades with alcohol or drugs. Once properly diagnosed and treated, these men and women return to health. Merely abstaining from the substance may have a negative effect on those suffering with a mental illness, if proper treatment of the illness is not received after detoxing. The self-medicating logic is that drugs or alcohol are medicine. For these men and women, drugs or alcohol is used to maintain a semi-normal life while coping with another illness that has gone unchecked.

Never be ashamed of seeking professional help. We must lose the thinking that we can address all issues simply because we offer a plan to live without substance dependence and or abuse/misuse. We here at Recovery 2-Day™ will never have all the solutions to your life's pressing issues. If someone uses our methods, then visited a licensed professional and never entered a meeting, he or she would be as successful as a person who came to a meeting just for information and got well.

These questions need to be answered honestly.

1.   Do you want to quit?
2.   Can you quit by yourself?
3.   Do you want to get well?

We have given you the medical tools used to diagnose abuse and dependence to determine the difference between abuse/misuse and dependence. We hope you are also clear on the fact that we do not want to strong-arm you. And in this, we started to develop the hope that climbs into a workable treatment plan.

1. Your treatment plan should show you the problem, factually.
2. Your treatment plan should help you, not degrade or define you.
3. Your treatment plan must be doable. We get well in degrees
4. Your treatment plan should not count time as success but you as the evidence of it.
5. Your treatment plan must be able to grow with you as you change.

RECOVERY 2-DAY™
IS BUILT TO DO THIS

THE ASCENT

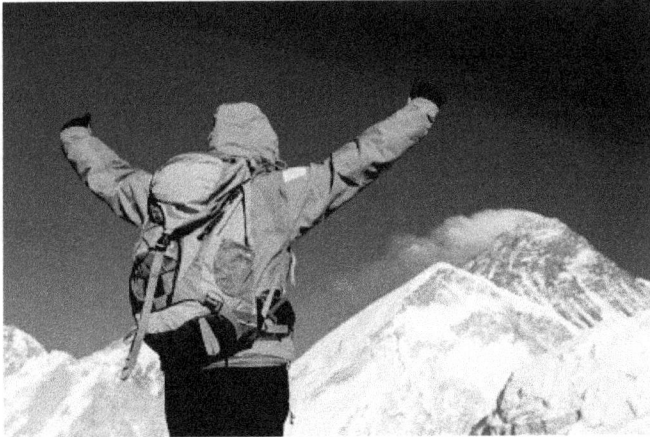

We left off the last chapter with a question Do you want to get well? You need to begin to see yourself as having the ability to get well.

To do this, you'll use a simple, but healthy, mental image of what getting well is going to entail. You start this with visual meditation. Visual meditation is very simple to grasp and to hold on to, even when the going gets hard. It is, in its basic form, a positive mental picture or self-image or goal. Your goal is to get well.

Your recovery journey to getting well starts by using the image of Mt. Everest. Each chapter going forward will use this metaphor with the symbolism of climbing up and down Mt Everest, the highest point on the planet. The climb is dangerous, exciting, rewarding, and can only be done by an individual. It is not easy for anyone. It is reproducible, but each time it will be different for anyone who attempts it. Experience is gained each day, both positive and negative. Courage is going to be tested, and every muscle of our bodies will be stressed. Lessons must be exact, since our life literally hangs on a knot.

If you cannot tie a proper knot in climbing, you jeopardize not only yourself but those who hang onto the same rope. This means it is not a time to experiment when being tutored, and it is not a time for a guide to experiment with the new climber being tutored. The basic elements must be covered in order for the new climber to find his or her own style later. But we never teach a personal style. We allow the next new climber to learn the basic knots, and then develop his or her own style without jeopardizing anyone else in the process. Hanging onto a rope means life and death. We want to know that the person who tied the knot is fully experienced and knows the gravity of the situation, and what is at stake. We will not gamble with your life.

There are so many parallels to recovery, and the climb that we believe it is helpful to everyone who attempts this. We must have an end in sight, a plan or goal. Our very simple goal is to get well, which is left open-ended, or undefined, for a reason. The degree of wellness you achieve will be the degree you earn by repeating certain things and gaining new tools on the way. Reaching the top is the goal. The top in our world is leaving substances for good and then learning how to live without them. After all, getting them out of our system, while painful, is the easy part, if a hospital or detox is used. Keeping them out and adjusting to life without them is hard.

Before anyone starts out to climb Mt. Everest, a team is put together. Those who come together to attempt the climb hire men and women as guides and muscle power. These are strong backs that will carry weeks of life-saving supplies, weather is considered, the variables change daily. Some days are better than others to climb, and even under the ideal conditions, many will not make it to the top.

Those who climb mountains hire help to carry the loads of equipment needed for success. They may spend thousands or climb on a budget. No one climbs for free. A price has to be paid to arrive, and the fee or license to climb Mt. Everest is ten thousand dollars, so it is not cheap to even dream of climbing it.

Our price, of course, is the years spent in abuse, the money, time, family etc., which have been lost. Some never to return. Human sacrifice is not new to the men and women that climb.

When groups decide to climb the tallest mountain in the world, a base camp is set up on arrival. Base camp is vital since that is where our life decisions will be defined. The most important decision will be which pass up Mt Everest will be taken.

The first lesson in our mountain-climbing example was, Who wants to climb with me? For us in Recovery 2-Day™, it will be Who wants to get well? Then each phase of climbing, from the initial plan to the end, is covered.

The parallels, we believe, are there. Life and death decisions are made daily; they start as soon as the climbers arrive at base camp. Who is the most experienced guide, the one who will make the team's calls when a decision must be made? An authority is needed to ensure success for the entire team. One of many or any of the decisions will or could determine success or failure for all in the group of climbers. Who ensures all the tools are in good working order before the climb is even started? Is anyone ever doomed to fail before they leave base camp, but they are simply too proud to stop?

Since weather plays such an important role daily, some days are not worth getting out of bed. Rest is needed, but energy is also needed at a moment's notice. But who can sleep in -35 degrees? The elements they face are harsh, cruel, and the slightest loss of focus does mean failure.

Climbers hire men, women, and even children to haul all their equipment, and then they climb, making stations at certain elevations. What many do not understand is that on the climb they actually climb down to rest, then climb higher once rested. This allows their bodies to get used to the higher elevations, without killing themselves in one straight upward climb. But on the final summit, they leave everything behind, even oxygen. The weight is too much to carry those last few feet. Driven by a purpose, they are willing to leave even the very thing they cannot live without to achieve their goal.

What is the lesson to learn from these climbers? First, they were driven by a purpose, a need to do something - at first a dream, then survival and an accomplishment that exceeds anyone's expectation. Once they have reached the top, they can mentally revisit the top, any time of any day for the rest of their lives.

Some might say, *Don't climb, since some die trying.* But if fear stopped them, they would have never gotten on the plane to attempt the climb. Make no mistake; fear is a daily companion that must be managed. Climbers must take satisfaction in that it has been done before and use that as part of the drive to succeed. I can do this must be part of their mindset.

Another clear and powerful message is how mountain climbers use others to lighten their load. They hire local men and women familiar with the terrain and elevations to help them carry their loads. No matter how strong they are or become, there are physical limits that must be observed. Here is where the value of people who rely on complete teams, hospitals, doctors, therapists, clergy, religion, self-determination, experience, knowledge, and some will take comfort in God to help carry their loads. Some do not believe in God, and will use those tools that they find best for them. No matter how they get there, the top will be the same, but the view is different for each climber.

The ascent has taken all the climbers have, especially on the final push. You would have had to endure the elements, from test of character, strength, personal convictions, courage, faith, sadness, grief, and doubt. You would have seen some fail; you have seen others succeed, only to face the end.

The end goal is to reach the top, and it must be done alone, without even the aid of oxygen. This type of effort explains why so few never make it to the top. To do so, they have to believe in themselves, and we will assume they have had to rely on a different kind of inner strength, as well. It would be very easy here to see that more than foxhole prayers are offered in this monumental human endeavor.

We watch so many try to climb a hill, the hill to recovery, and they act as if they alone are to push their load up that hill, carrying all the burdens of life with them. Our minds paint a picture of the mythological Sisyphus, sentenced to an eternity of pushing a huge boulder up a hill, only for it to roll back down again. This struggle is frustrating, to say the least, and is repeated over and over again. These people either seek help or give up. We know how hard it is to ask for help, but to be successful, we must have help in those first days. The burden, of course, is the physical and emotional damage from years of past abuse.

But the professional mountain climber hires someone to carry his or her load. That they are smart enough to ask for help is another lesson. They also watched the weather and on days that it was too difficult to climb, they rested and tried again the next day. They actually used the experience of those who had gone before – yet another lesson. They used the authority of others to help them become authorities themselves. They used the latest technologies available, and nothing is left to chance. The more they climbed, the better they became at climbing. They accepted the fact that climbing down was part of climbing up. This required dedication and years of training.

No one is foolish enough to take on Mt. Everest on day one. Each climber had to start on lower elevations, and as they progressed to the top, they had to learn to breathe at each new elevation. It was critical for them to be acclimated before they could proceed higher and higher.

Once their brains, lungs, and bodies were trained, they had to learn all the tools, knots, clips, and gear. They were almost there. Then they hired guides to help climb the mountain. And when they got to nearly the top, they removed all the weight to make the final summit.

Our journey into recovery can be seen at each stage of climbing Mt. Everest. At each stage of progress, from base camp, to Camp 2, then on to Camp 3, time is spent on each level. The lungs need get used to the higher elevations. Then the climbers make the ascent, and as quickly as they make the final top, they must descend.

Your progress is similar. Each new tool you learn in recovery must be practiced before you move on, but your tools must be practiced in unison with the other tools. You need to become the complete climber, not a part-timer, so that recovery becomes instinctive, almost involuntary like breathing or blinking your eyes. It is not habit. It is a practice. When a daily practice is experienced, it becomes a natural reflex. Sometimes, an hourly practice each day dictates which tools are needed.

There are also groups of people who come to watch. They gather at the base of Mt. Everest and watch the climbers. Some critique the climbers, some pull for favorites, and some are fans, never leaving the safety of their chair.

Last, but not least, when the ascent is finished, the descent is quick, and the climbers do not pick up the supplies they carried up the mountain. They leave them all behind, again using the hired help to carry their burdens. They leave the mountain with the vision they have seen at the top of the world.

Not everyone who tries makes it to the top. Some never get in shape to make the ascent. Some are injured on the way. Some say they are ready, when they have merely tied a knot once. The worst thing a guide can allow to happen is to place an amateur on a crest too high to climb.

Some of the men and women climbers return to act as guides for those who have never made the climb. The guide does not carry the new climber to the top, since that would be impossible. If the weight of an oxygen bottle were too heavy, to carry the weight of another would kill both of them. But these experienced guides can show climbers the way.

Trust is required. You must determine who your authority is and do as they tell you, until you have mastered the lesson. Once that lesson is learned, you can adapt it to your own style. Show me, is the lesson you must demand of your guides in order to place your trust in them. If you cannot tie the knot, you cannot teach anyone to tie it properly.

There are many people who never climb the mountain, but they speak as if they have, since they have watched others do it. Or maybe they have read a book with pictures and can describe it in detail, but have no clue what they are saying. These types are the most dangerous because a new climber may follow their advice and die using a path no one ever attempted but sounded as if they had.

The image of climbing Mt. Everest will be our method to describe the process of how to get well. It's our climb from dependence to success. Success will be your ability to not only avoid future episodes of drugs or alcohol abuse or dependence, but being able to help others achieve the same goal.

We did not choose the symbol of Mt. Everest at random. Visually we need a positive reinforcement that is easy to grasp, and attach to mentally. The idea of a climb is accurate, and the different elevations are very similar to the process of getting well. *Wellness comes in degrees* or when new ideas and growth happens.

BASE CAMP
WHICH PASS TO TAKE?

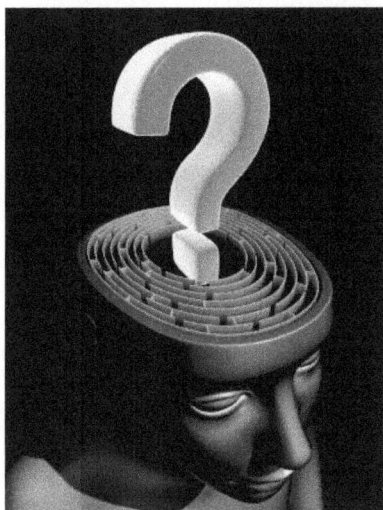

There are four sides to consider when climbing Mt. Everest: East, West, North and South passes. Only one person has climbed all four.

There are two passes most climb today, both tried and proven with reproducible success: the North Pass and the South Pass. We use the metaphor of climbing Mt Everest for this reason. The South Pass plan, outlined in Recovery 2-Day™ combines cognitive tools and spiritual tools that are of help for those that believe in a God.

The North Pass plan combines cognitive and meditation tools, that omit terms such as God or prayer.

Having two editions or plans/passes offers you the choice, so you don't have to read around words that would or could otherwise make you leave. Now you see why our name has a 2 in it. It represents choice.

Deciding which pass to climb will dictate the proper gear you need, a starting point will tell you where to begin the climb. Your guide will show you what is needed each day.

At the Base Camp the climbers decide who is going to climb the North Pass and who is going to climb the South Pass.

Both passes have warning pages, so that your personal beliefs are not challenged by having to read around words you may not believe in.

To keep the entrance simple, we have created equal tools for separate groups. To respect both groups we created two separate recovery paths.

For any atheists or agnostics where terms such as God or prayer are offensive or against their beliefs, we created the North Pass tools, where we speak freely of those beliefs.

For those who believe in a Theos, Deity, God, gods, of any religions, the South Pass is created where words such as God, prayer are used where we speak freely, of those beliefs.

As a helpful guide, we use this legend:

[P] Prayer (used in South Pass only)
[M] Meditation (used in both)
[T] Thinking (cognitive skills, contemplation)

In each pass, the [P] or [M] or [T] Legend will be shown beside something we are to [P] pray about, [M] meditate about or [T] contemplate. When you see this in the next chapters, it is telling you: *I should [P] pray here, or I should [M] meditate here or [T] consider this.*

RECOVERY 2 DAY™
NORTH PASS ENTRANCE

FOR THOSE WHO PREFER THAT TERMS SUCH AS 'GOD' OR 'PRAYER' ARE NOT USED IN THEIR TREATMENT PLAN.

FROM BASE CAMP TO CAMP 1,
CAMP 1 - NORTH PASS

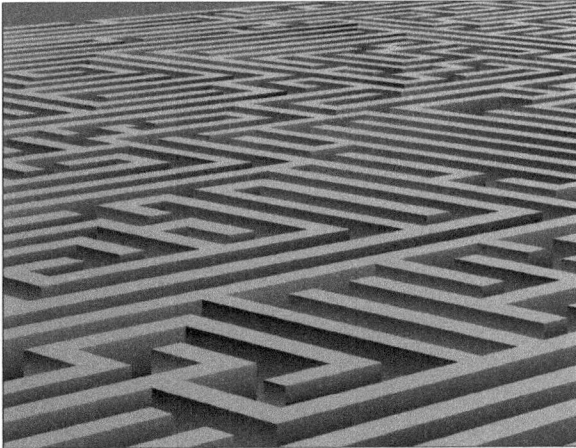

Those people who had common sense and personal endurance discovered the North Pass of Mt Everest. They knew that there had to be more than one way to scale a mountain. The reason we needed to create our North Pass Edition is that simple. Since chemical dependence is a disease, we had to create a treatment plan for men and women who did not want or need theism-based "higher power" transference.

Previously we described what neurobiologists have medically established: that prolonged chemical use causes neurotransmitter dysregulation, which is a brain disease. Because of this diagnosis, we can now move forward in its treatment. Prior to this, books and articles written about abuse or dependence have rarely treated it as a real medical condition. Research has shown that misuse of a substance can lead to dependence in some people. Many treat their problems by self-medicating, which may soon shift to meet the criterion of abuse, combating or creating maladaptive behaviors. Once dysregulation occurs, the criterion of chemical dependence is met.

Over the past ten years, science has consistently made advances in the treatment of receptor uptake sites. Understanding serotonin and how it can be used in the treatment of depression is an excellent example. Pharmacologists are making breakthroughs daily. During detoxifications medicines are used today to help a person avoid withdrawals or seizures, valuable techniques that have advanced through scientific research. When we connect this with cognitive therapy, we have a winning solution to recovery from misuse, abuse, and dependence. Combining this knowledge with our own and others' past experiences has allowed Recovery 2 Day™ to develop a new choice in the recovery industry. We believe that merging the sciences makes complete sense for the recovery industry. *Which brings us to today. Now a substance problem no longer has to be treated as something that requires a moral or religious conversion.* Until Recovery 2 Day™, an agnostic or atheist who suffered from a substance problem had little choice in the treatment prescribed by the self-help recovery industry.

We begin the North Pass with an apology to all of you who feel you have been abused or mistreated by a religion or self-help group that promotes a Theos to treat a disease. No other diagnosed disease is medically treated this way! We feel it is important to offer an apology to all agnostics and atheists. It is an apology made out of respect to you, and we feel that it is long overdue.

We are so sorry that this has happened to you.

The agnostic and atheist have historically received the harshest treatment when they have sought help for their substance-abuse problems. Many have had their beliefs severely questioned or have had to hide them. Or they've been forced to tolerate various religious practices that are not a part of their personal beliefs.

For the past few decades most inpatient and outpatient state-funded treatment centers had little choice but to send their clients to fellowship meetings, established by various faith based self-help recovery networks. To be in or out of compliance of a treatment plan, rarely took into consideration a person's religious beliefs. Once a person was labeled as either an addict or an alcoholic, they were regarded as not having the ability to make good decisions. Consequently, they were easily abused or manipulated to succumb to other peoples' religion or faith. For many years, there was not another option of places to send someone with a substance problem.

What happens to a person who does not believe in that flavor of treatment? What happens to someone who finds it impossible to pray for help to a God they don't believe in? The substance problem remains untreated. Meanwhile they are bombarded with critical and judgmental remarks such as, "This is what we do" and "if you do not like it, leave." The issue obviously is that, upon leaving treatment, the underlying problem is still left untreated. The person who sought help finds that their feelings of fear, anger, and hopelessness have escalated. This helps explain why so many older disease theories, that maintain chemical dependence is a spiritual disease, have such low success rates with agnostics and atheists. If a person holding different beliefs does not conform to the majority self-help group philosophy, he or she can feel unwelcome. The prevailing attitude in the self-help groups towards agnostics and atheists traditionally is that they have not suffered enough to convert, but that day will come. It's as if a good dose of fear will straighten them out and eventually they will comply. If a person does not believe in the conversion concept, they are made to feel unwelcome, even though they have no problem accepting the truth that they have a problem. Much like the guest of a country club, they are only welcome at the behest of the member. Equal rights, or freedom from religion, is not offered. Sometimes the terms such as "higher power" and "God are interchangeable, but the fact is that they are referring to the same thing. Most agnostics and atheists are not fooled by syntax, vernacular, and subjective interpretation. This is not choice as we see it. It remains, "convert or be excommunicated."

Several state supreme courts have ruled on this freedom from religion issue, making it one of the most important issues in many areas of our lives. The North Pass edition of Recovery 2 Day™ was created out of our firm conviction in the importance of freedom from religion. It exists for all those men and women who seek a treatment plan for their substance problem that does not require a religious conversion, religious practices of prayer or worship, spiritual experience or spiritual awakening. Instead, their treatment plan is based in current science, cognitive and behavioral methodology, common sense, and real-life experience. Cognitive therapy is a common sense approach to problem solving. By solving one problem, that same methodology can be transferred to other life issues. This sets the stage perhaps to solve other problems as they appear to us by trial and error, and experimentation. You will start to see the value of *adaptability*, you learn to mold the tools to suit your individual needs. The severity of your problems are of course complex and completely subjective to you the owner of the problem at hand. This makes it perfectly clear, that the solutions to these problems remain in eye of the beholder. Once one problem is solved, you use the same tools, in future problems, by gaining confidence in your own abilities, you develop your self-esteem. For all future needs or problems, the tools learned here, allows you to determine which is more of a priority and focuses your attention on what bothers you the most. Having the success of solving the first problem, allows you to gain confidence in solving other issues as the crop up.

Recovery 2 Day™ North Pass edition begins by asking you this one question: *Do you think you have a problem?* Notice we use the term **problem**, which covers the wide range of problems we all must face. But there's one that affects every other problem you might be having. Substance abuse affects you emotionally, mentally, and physically. How you can maintain a life free from your substance problem and *stay free* is the purpose of this book.

This is done by helping you connect to your basic human cognitive emotions and, using the North Pass tools, showing you how to manage them.

Once the North Pass tools are outlined and understood, we outline a plan specifically designed for you. Recovery 2 Day™ makes one promise to you: *You get well in degrees.*

CLIMBING TO CAMP 2

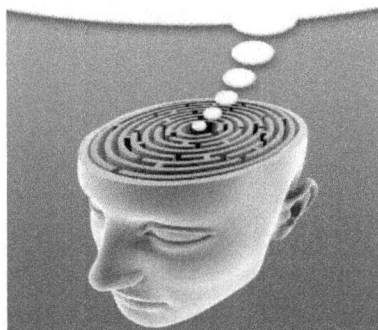

When a person climbing Mt. Everest suffers from hypothermia, which is a sudden drop in body temperature, scant minutes can make the difference between life and death. If left untreated, this dangerous drop in body temperature can kill a person in thirty minutes. Another challenge of climbing Mt. Everest can be frostbite, where body parts sometimes freeze and break off. Even if you survive frostbite, the full extent of the damage may not be known for up to six months later.

Climbers of Mt. Everest face exposure to jet winds of up to 95 MPH and sub-zero temperatures as low as -33 degrees. Makes climbing your own personal Mt. Everest inside yourself seem a bit less daunting, doesn't it? On the other hand, it does explain why so very few attempt this amazing feat of human endurance.

Just as with a real climb up Mt. Everest, the beginning of your adventure in Recovery 2-Day is the hardest part. You will not face hypothermia. You will face yourself, and what weight of your past and present that you carry. Just like the person who suffers from hypothermia, you are fighting for survival. You cannot waste time in the recovery room. You do not have the luxury of magical thinking until you feel better. It has to happen now. Today. You need to quickly learn how to press on, despite your initial misgivings that perhaps this is impossible.

We hear two common excuses used when men and women enter recovery, I don't want to rush into anything, and I'm not there yet. Throw that logic out the window *now*. Replace it with the idea that you cannot waste a minute! You must start immediately!

Short-Lists

As we said, this initial part of Recovery 2-Day is the most difficult. The cognitive skills you'll learn here are called *Short-Lists*.

We use the terms Short-Lists and Short-Listing wisely, the names used in our naming convention, describes the mechanical process. Common sense rules, you will create "short" cognitive lists. These Short-Lists will be addressing your basic human emotions, *Anger, Fear and Security*. Notice also the term "security" instead of love you will see them both, *love and security* used synonymously.

Learn them well. If you practice Short-Listing on a daily basis, they will serve you for the rest of your life. Each skill is practical and easy to use, but sometimes painful in the beginning, as you begin to see things as they really are. The skills you learn here need to be seen as part of something that will be much bigger when you are finished. Much like a chain on a bike, each tool you are given here at Recovery 2-Day is a vital part of the overall skills program, but each individual part is needed to make up the whole bike or plan. Without the chain, the bike will not work.

Short-Listing Anger

Anger is the first emotion we list, and the easiest to address.

Here are the directions for listing our anger in order to manage anger instead of anger managing us. **Take a pen, or pencil and a few pieces of paper.** However, before you start, we will offer a few guiding thoughts. This is not a test. No one will see this list when you are finished. If you want to burn your anger list when you are done, that is your decision. Make sure you dispose of it safely. (We must also point out that illegal activities listed would be seen as a legal confession in a court of law and, yes, held against you. This is not legal counsel but common sense. Keep your anger list in a safe place, safe from eyes that could hurt you with it.)

You are far more prone to drink or drug when you're feeling anger or fear, since these are your weakest moments. If you have a tool for managing anger and fear, it makes sense that you would stand a much better defense against taking the first drug or drink going forward. This will attach to the other cognitive tools you have been introduced to: Stroop charts, Stop sign, and Eye Movement Movement Desensitization and Reprocessing (EMDR).

The best way to do this is to create quick, short lists every day. The good thing about short lists is that they deal with only your most current problems, as they exist today. Since each day is different, each short list will show you how your emotions affect you.

When emotions affect you, you feel, and then you act on that feeling, which is called your behavior. In a straight line, it looks like this: thinking→ feelings→ behaviors. Simple, right?

Anger is a critical emotion that drives your feelings, which causes you to act or behave a certain way.

The name of the Short-Lists tool is self-descriptive: Make short lists. *Long lists are overwhelming and will delay your progress.* The name itself, *Short- Listing,* defines the skill you'll be developing. Later it will be addressed as What bothered me 2-Day? You need to *learn* how to do this, and do this daily. This is your map up the mountain, which will serve you for the rest of your life. *You learn this in a day and practice it for a lifetime.* You need to be fully committed to the journey. It starts now.

This is one of the biggest differences you'll find in our recovery philosophy. Most self-help groups believe that "it takes months to do this." At Recovery 2 Day™ our motto is: **Learn this in a day, practice it for a lifetime.**

Here's an example: A woman attending a self-help group was describing how our learn this in a day philosophy had been so helpful to her. Now she practices it easily and does it in minutes each day.

A person who had been attending self-help groups for many years, abruptly stated, *"It takes months or years to do that!"* He could not understand how this young woman could become so healthy so quickly.

The woman replied honestly, *"I did not have years – or even months."* She needed immediate relief. Her words showed clearly that had she sat doing nothing or waited for someone else's permission to get well, it would have been too late. , She could not afford the option of magical thinking. Her only option was to start getting well *today.*

One of the basic cognitive elements of Recovery 2-Day is for you to keep the process simple by only dealing with what is current, or what is bothering you *right now.* Ask yourself: Is it happening *now,* in this moment? This is the day you need to get well. 2-Day. Our name, Recovery 2-Day is the reason we say constantly, You are in Recovery 2-Day.

This means you are getting better each moment. In Recovery 2-Day you are not waiting for something to happen or someone's permission to proceed. You are getting better *now*.

Since no one is going to see your list, besides yourself, be honest. *No one has done this perfectly, so you will not be the first.*

Now pick up the pen and start. Create a short current list of people you are angry at, including institutions or concepts. If you are angry with yourself, reserve that spot for last. You will take care of that in Camp 3, the next elevation of your daily climb. Remember, you are not looking for a complete history. You just want a short list. It's a list that can be managed 2-Day.

Now and then, we've met a person who believes, "I'm not angry with anything, or anyone." If you feel this way too, instead of forcing the issue, start your *Short List* by writing out your Fears, which we describe in the next section. You can return to the anger list after you've worked on your short fears list. Most of the time, it simply takes a bit of loosening up for us to see the emotion anger in its proper light. The point is not to haggle over which came first: the anger or the fear.

Take comfort in the knowledge you are not in trouble for feeling this way. Nevertheless, feeling this way may cause you trouble.

What does this list look like? See **Example Q1**. Notice it is short and current: it only lists what the person was angry at today.

As you write your list, make sure you have committed to being honest with yourself. Be as honest as you can be. You get well in degrees, and this also means the more you practice this, the more self-honesty you receive and practice.

Warning: Do not shortchange yourself by not writing this out on a piece of paper. It makes an important difference to face your emotional truths line by line, honestly.

The Short-List of Anger Questions **Q1-Q5** are simple. They are as follows:

Q1: Who am I mad at 2-Day?
Q2: Briefly, why am I mad at them or it?
Q3: How does this make me feel?
Q4: How long have I held these thoughts or feelings?
Q5: Do I like feeling this way?

Example Q1,
Who am I mad at 2-Day?

My Mother

My Father

Spouse or partner

Religious people

My Boss

The Judge

Person in Junior High school

You'll see that the examples are referred to by numbers. **Example Q1** demonstrates how you begin an Anger List. You make a vertical list of people, institutions, or principles with which you have current, burning issues, feel anger toward, or even hatred. You deal only with the now. In Example **Q1**, it listed My Mother and continued down listing the current Who am I angry with 2-Day.

After listing five or ten current events, return to the top of your list. Starting with the first person on the list, move over and create another column titled:

Why?

If you feel stuck, ;ook at Example **Q2** to get some ideas.

In a few words or less, list the reason you are mad at the person, institution, or principle on the list. If one word reminds you of why you are mad, one word is enough. This is where most people want to spend a long time, trying to explain in detail all the injuries and injustices done to them. But keep this brief. This is not a writing contest.

In Example **Q2**, the person is mad at his mother for saying to him at the age of six, "I wish you had never been born." Once that reason is listed – no matter how painful! – simply continue on to the next person, listing one by one, why you are angry with them.

Directions: Go to the top of your list after looking at Example **Q2** and fill out the **Why** section against each item on your list. Be honest and use as few words as possible to give the necessary information. In other words, be brief. It is important here that you write in a "north south, top to bottom manner, try to **avoid the tendency of writing** *left to right or right to left* since the list reveals information as you write, patterns start to reveal themselves if done properly. By writing from left to right, it is more difficult to see your patterns if you write side to side, "left to right or right to left," since we tend to only focus on the one item, instead of the entire list.

Example Q2, Briefly, Why am I mad at them or it?

Short-List	Why (briefly)
My Mother	told me she wished I'd never been born when I was six
My Father	left when I was six
Spouse or partner	left me over my drugs and alcohol, said she hated me
Religious people	deny science and education, intolerant, self righteous, fanatics
My Boss	fired me for stealing, never trusted me
The Judge	Sentenced me to rehab
Person in Junior High school	called me a name

With two columns completed as shown in **Example Q2**, you must do three more things; first, you must now ask certain questions about each person on your list.

Now return to the top of your list and start to find out how this anger affected your feelings. About each person listed, ask yourself a series of questions. You can take ideas from the **Example Q2**, and use this partial list of feelings:

Insecure	Embarrassed
Sad	Guilty
Disconnected	Anxious
Prideful	Jealous
Envious	Obsessed
Lonely	Superior
Inferior	Threatened
Betrayed	Lost
Overwhelmed	Confused

Did the anger with your mother make you feel insecure? If yes, write down "insecure." This creates **Example Q3.**

Did the anger with your mother make you feel embarrassed? If yes, list it. The list of questions is used for each person/institution you listed.

Did this anger make me feel___? (fill in question with list below) If yes, write how it makes or made you feel, beside the person name.

Warning: The temptation may be to discount your feelings, and not write them or to shorten the list by using abbreviations (like writing "INS" as a shorthand code for "INSecure"). This may appear to make your journey faster going, but there are no short cuts while climbing Mt. Everest.

Reminder: Keep it simple. Short lists are more manageable, less overwhelming, and still produce the desired results. You'll find you have a completed list in minutes, not days or weeks. It outlines your current life situations, not your complete life, but your largest challenges, because they're coming at you right now. 2-Day. Your current moment is sitting in front of you, facing you.

Example Q3	Why (briefly)	Q3 Made me feel?
My Mother	*told me she wished I'd never been born when I was six*	**Insecure, sad, guilty, embarrassed, fearful, disconnected, jealous envy, pride, anxious, threatened, lonely**
My Father	*left when I was six*	**Insecure, sad, guilty, embarrassed, fearful, disconnected, jealous envy, pride, anxious, threatened, lonely**
Spouse or partner	*left me over my drugs and alcohol, said "she hated me"*	**Sad, guilty, jealous, threatened, anxious, insecure, embarrassed, inferior**
Religious people	*deny science and education, intolerant, self righteous, fanatics*	Guilty, ashamed, embarrassed, doubtful, fearful, disconnected, inferior, sad, superior
My Boss	*fired me for stealing, never trusted me*	**Insecure, sad, superior, inferior, anxious, jealous, guilty, embarrassed**
The Judge	*Sentenced me to rehab*	**Inferior, embarrassed, guilty, anxious, jealous**
Person in Junior High school	*called me a name*	**Embarrassed, insecure, sad, jealous**

Before continuing your climb, pause here and look at the list you have just written Consider it carefully, as though you're looking at the view around you. Look at the effect on you of being angry at whoever is on your list. It is worth taking this time to examine the effects of anger in your daily life.

If you have been honest, this list will tell you a lot about yourself. Now, relax, nothing has changed. You still may hate them, you are still mad at them. Maybe now that you've written out the 'why', you feel even more justified in feeling angry.

Anger makes you very predictable. You may not like to hear that. But have you ever wondered why certain people always push your buttons? It is because you have those buttons hanging off your clothes to push, and quite easily, too.

Nothing has changed is the most obvious result right now if you are staring at your list of people or events with whom you are angry. The longer you pause and review the list, it seems the worse the list looks. Perhaps you are feeling uncomfortable, madder even, since listing this has brought up your past. Looking at it makes you relive it, and it hurts all over again.

If done as we outlined it, you landed exactly where we wanted you to land, so good job! (And if it just upset you that we predicted this, it will not be the first time we have ended up on someone's list).

But if you stay here, nothing will change, and you will die from exposure. So it's okay to feel mad.

Two more questions need to be asked about your current list. How many years have you carried this burden? Remember the image of a person trying to push a boulder up a hill, only to have it roll back over him, so he gives up or gets help?

Try to put an estimate of the number of years you have been angry with each person on your anger list. Look at your list and try to determine this.

Q4: How long have I held these thoughts or feelings?

Example 1.4:	How Long?	Why (briefly)	Made me feel?
My Mother	**26 yrs**	*told me she wished I'd never been born when I was six*	*Insecure, sad, guilty, embarrassed, fearful, disconnected, jealous envy, pride, anxious, threatened, lonely*
My Father	**26 yrs**	*left when I was six*	*Insecure, sad, guilty, embarrassed, fearful, disconnected, jealous envy, pride, anxious, threatened, lonely*
Spouse or partner	**5 yrs**	*left me over my drugs and alcohol, said she hated me*	*Sad, guilty, jealous, threatened, anxious, insecure, embarrassed, inferior*
Religious people	**21 yrs**	*deny science and education, intolerant, self righteous, fanatics*	*Guilty, ashamed, embarrassed, doubtful, fearful, disconnected*
My Boss	**8 yrs**	*fired me for stealing, never trusted me*	*Insecure, sad, superior, inferior, anxious, jealous, guilty, embarrassed*
The Judge	**2 yrs**	*Sentenced me to rehab*	*Inferior, embarrassed, guilty, anxious, jealous*
Person in Junior High school	**31 yrs**	*called me a name*	*Embarrassed, insecure, sad, jealous*

In Example **Q4**, we see the first person on the list is the writer's mother. This event happened when he was six years old. When he created this list for the first time, he was 32, which tells us this event was carried for 26 years. This means that the event has flowed through many years and many failed relationships.

In other words, this even has replayed in this person's mind millions of times. The weight is crushing. Can you hear the voices? "I wish I would have said, I could have said, I should have said, I could have done, why did it happen?" The fact that his mother is the one who hurt him makes it even worse. This one anger event is revisited over and over; the flames reignite with each visit or thought. This person is constantly reliving the past.

Most of us spend our entire lives this way, living in the past, but hardly realizing how heavily it weighs on us. When we add the years in all the blocks together, do they not span our entire lives?

How much weight do you think you can carry?

Q5: Review List - Do I like feeling this way?

Example	How Long?	Why (briefly)	Made me feel?
			Insecure, sad, guilty, embarrassed, fearful, disconnected, jealous, envy, pride, **anxious**, threatened, lonely
			Insecure, sad, guilty, embarrassed, fearful, disconnected, jealous, envy, pride, **anxious**, threatened, lonely
Q5: Do I like feeling this way?			Sad, guilty, jealous, threatened, **anxious**, **insecure**, embarrassed, inferior
			Guilty, ashamed, embarrassed, doubtful, fearful, disconnected
			Insecure, sad, superior, inferior, **anxious**, jealous, guilty, embarrassed
			Inferior, embarrassed, guilty, **anxious**, jealous
			Embarrassed, **insecure**, sad, jealous

We believe a person who enters the world of substance dependence can endure more emotional pain than anyone can imagine.

What else does your list show? Can you start to see how being angry cuts you consciously off from life, from almost everything you love? Can you see that while you are angry, it is impossible to feel mentally connected and in control? Is it not more important to have peace, than to be cut off? Can you see how you let anger dominate us? Is this what is meant by "peace of mind"?

Your next task is to cover the first three columns with a piece of paper, as in **Example Q5**. While you have the first three columns covered, consider how your anger has affected all areas of your personal feelings about yourself. This is question, *Q5: "Do I like feeling this way?"*

Now look at your list with the first three columns covered. See what happens if you mentally exchange the person on the bottom with the person on the middle, and the person in the middle with the person on the top. Imagine dropping the first three columns on the floor like a deck of cards, and shuffling them. You'll find that the emotions or "made me feel column" are the same.

In each case, the person or persons that you listed have affected all areas of our emotional lives, from insecurities to sadness, guilt to envy, and so on.

You will start to see that it is the thought or "rethinking" of the anger event that is driving the feelings you hold. You start to see that how you think about a person or thing and how you attach in your memories the feelings to people, is driving your behavior towards that person and to everyone else around us.

Do you find that amazing? Because it is. There is really no difference between the person who hit you in junior high and your hurtful mother, since both people create the same feeling of anger.

Your anger is what makes you feel insecure, sad, guilty, envious, etc., and affects your sense of pride and well-being.

Therefore, *angry thoughts, not people, are what dominate you.* It's time to learn how to live with the effects of anger so that they don't affect you any longer. "Impossible," you say, —and it's true that this is very difficult. But you can do it.

At this stage, you won't be able to live without anger, but you're already well on your way to the place where you truly can. To be free you need to learn how to release this emotion in the proper way. Some anger can fall from us simply by listing it "cognitive awareness." Other things that have lingered for longer periods will need treatment, of a special kind.

So how do we manage our anger?

Before we cover that, if you will recall, we also listed another emotion, Fear. Can you have anger without fear?

Yes.

Can you have anger and fear with the same event?

Of course, you can. Often you are so wrapped up in your anger that you don't realize that your fear is never far away. These two emotions wrapped together are often called the fight or flight response. We either react or we run.

At Recovery 2-Day™ it's called the knee jerk response. If someone says something you do not like, you react immediately. Most of the time you may not even know why you react the way you do. Different issues affect everyone differently; however, everyone has a reaction.

If you feel threatened, you typically react with either anger or fear. These two emotions tend to dominate all the others. Think of the classic story of Pinocchio, the story of a puppet boy made of wood, with strings attached to make him move. Imagine the strings are your emotions and feelings. People pull your strings, and your knee jerks. Other terms for the same idea are: "push my buttons" or "get on my last nerve."

So how do you cut the strings so that you're free to move on your own? The first way is by learning the cognitive skill of "short-listing."

The next step is to treat the anger with awareness and meditation. By combining cognitive skills with meditation, you're on your path to recovery 2-day.

Anger and fear are always going to present themselves. But by learning how to practice meditation, you'll learn a skill that will help you manage your anger and your fear. Learning how to manage your anger will be a tool for life.

A common and tragic truth in the lives of dependence or abuse is that many of us are victims of violent crimes, rape, incest, violence, and murder. If you have people listed who brought these crimes into your life, it will appear natural to hate them. Nothing that you're learning here is making an excuse for those tragic events.

But with practice you can set yourself free from your anger and fear, and you can get well.

Before we continue, allow us to say to you sincerely and heartfelt, *I am so deeply sorry this happened to you. It should have never happened.*

The people who harmed you are sick emotionally and mentally and need help. But you need to get better and leave those feelings and events where they belong - in the past. Trauma events are best dealt with by the help of medical professionals, and may require long-term therapy.

Hating people who harmed you will only delay your return to health, since hate and anger are the chain that keeps you locked in the past.

A forgiveness meditation helps to release them from your mind so that you can move forward.

For those of you who have never learned to meditate: here is a brief introduction: Breathing is used to relax you into a state of mind that is calm and reflective. (See the chapter Going Solo In Meditation if you are not comfortable with this and return here after reading those directions).

To begin, find a comfortable chair to sit in, close your eyes, and exhale. If an image of someone comes to your mind, or you experience a feeling of anxiousness as you breathe out, imagine yourself exhaling the feelings. If you have an image of a person frozen in your thoughts, close your eyes, and use the eye movement technique to unlock it or begin again by using the Stroop chart.

With your eyes closed go to your safe place mentally, imagine its textures, imagine its smells, relax into your safe place, breathe in, breathe out, breathe in, breathe out, and relax.

Take your list and cover it, showing only the names we listed 2-Day.

See **Example 1.6**.

Now you are looking at the list of people you hate or are angry with currently 2-Day.

Now as you meditate, forgive everyone on this list, one at time. Short-listing is a daily habit, as was said earlier. You're not going to stop with just making your lists. You're also going to learn to meditate over them.

Example 1.6

My Mother

My Father

Spouse or partner

Religious people

My Boss

The Judge
Person in Junior High school

Use **Example 1.6** as your guideline. Your list will have different names attached. Now use meditation to move through each person or thing on your Short List of Anger.

Directions: [M] While in your safe place, bring into your mind, the image of the first person on your list, exhale, breathe, now in your mind say, "I forgive you, Mother." After a moment you might want to add these words: "I forgive you for anything you may have done in the past, either intentionally or unintentionally, through your thoughts, words, or actions, that caused me pain. I forgive you." Now, release the image of that person in your mind. Note: This is not condoning a person who has harmed you; it is releasing you from the burden they have caused you to carry.

To move to the next person on the list, you need to clear your mind of the image you left behind. To do this, use your eye movement tool (EMDR).

Close your eyelids, then move your eyes, as if you are looking down hard right. Keeping your eyelids closed, look hard left. Repeat this three times. Then open your eyes.

Now move to the next person on your list.

And again,

[M] While in your safe place, bring into your mind the image of the next person on your list. Exhale, breathe, now in your mind say "I forgive you, Father." "I forgive you for anything you may have done in the past, either intentionally or unintentionally, through your thoughts, words, or actions, that caused me pain. I forgive you." Now, release the image of him in your mind.

To move to the next person on the list, you first need to clear your mind of the image of that person you just forgave. To do this, again use your eye movement tool.

Close your eyelids, now move your eyes, as if you are looking down hard right, then keeping your eyelids closed, look hard left, and repeat this three times. Then open your eyes.

Now move to the next person on the list.

Use this technique for each person or thing on your list. You'll be amazed how it works to begin to free you from the chains of anger and fear right away.

Here is a blank example

[M] **Bring into your mind, the image of the first person on your list, exhale, breathe, and now in your mind say "I forgive you <u>Fill-in the Blank</u>. I forgive you for anything you may have done in the past, either intentionally or unintentionally, through your thoughts, words, or actions that caused me pain. I forgive you."**

Now, release the image of that person in your mind. Close your eyelids, now move your eyes, as if you are looking down hard right, then keeping your eyelids closed, look hard left, and repeat this three times. Then open your eyes.

Repeat this practice until you have offered forgiveness over every person on your list. Skip one here and you may not get well, since you are still trying to carry this burden up the mountain. Have you not carried this long enough?

Note to Guides: if you are guiding someone through this forgiveness meditation, see the instructions for leading focused meditation and do not violate a person's safe place.

It is important to do this over each person on the list individually. This is not a blanket meditation to be said over the page of names, but single simple visual images that you can see and hold and then release.. People learn best by repetition, and this repetition creates a tool, a skill set. The repeated use of focused meditation becomes a natural process for your future recovery.

Sometimes at this moment you may have what is called an *aha moment*, an uplifting of your consciousness, or real sense of release. The calm you feel, in that moment, may feel profound. Don't be upset if you wake up the next day feeling mad at the very same people you *Short Listed* hours before. The process repeats itself; make a new *Short List*, listing what is bothering you 2 day, etc... Meditate over the same things as the day before and, in time, you will find that the person or thing will not return to the *Short List*. Some events are released in moments, some take weeks, or months to remove.

Remember how many years you spent carrying your burdens, the burdens of anger on the list you just made? Your journey is a process. By starting today, and staying with it, you will get better – and you will stay better.

Thus starts the process of our daily *Short Listing*. A quick list of five to ten people is all you need to start and is much less overwhelming to look at. Short lists are the most effective. They relieve your emotional pressure at a much safer rate. Remember, you get well in degrees.

Returning to Mt. Everest for a moment, on the climb to Camp 2, a person's lungs must acclimate, or get used to the lack of oxygen at each elevation they reach. Your quick Short Lists do the same. Depending on the person, this practice of Short Listing needs to done daily for at least three weeks for it to become habit, a very good one. Meditation is a skill that requires practice and the rewards – peace, health, a sense of well-being – are indescribable.

If you've carried a burden for many years, living free from them is sometimes as difficult as living with them. Every day you are going to have to readjust your load, as it grows lighter.

Imagine being able to manage anger--or at least being able to understand how it affects you, and the years of trouble it has caused you.

You're going to leave all your burdens on the mountain. Your daily listing is the way to unload your burdens. If you have carried a burden for 20 or 30 years, and then it is removed, it takes time to find your balance without the weight of the anger you once felt. As crazy as it sounds, you are used to living angry. All you have to do is look at your list to show you how long it has been carried. Study the question **Q5:** "Do you like feeling this way?" reveals a lot about our self.

Despite this, it may tempting to put those burdens back on again. You may be more comfortable feeling the weight of your burden than not having them. You have actually gotten used to living with your burden, strange, as it seems. Living without them is almost unthinkable. What will you do without them? Freedom can be just as scary as bondage, if not more so, since it is very unfamiliar at first.

Now take a deep breath. Before you move on to your next list, look at the anger list once more. Have you treated these people on your list the way you have been treated or the way you would like to be treated? Your families, have you been honest with them? Your employers, have you been the best employees you could be?

Example 1.2	Why (briefly)	Made me feel?
	told me she wished I'd never been born when I was six	
	left when I was six	
	left me over my drugs and alcohol, said she hated me	
	I lived a life I am ashamed of and scared I was bad, feel like I can't be forgiven	
	fired me for stealing, never trusted me	
	sentenced me to rehab	
	called me a name	

If you had a time machine, like the science fiction movies that go back in time, would you do anything differently?

It is normal at this stage of the process for you to feel regrets and remorse. But keep in mind that you want to get well. You do not return to those old days, months or years that were lost to anger? These glimpses of self-honesty are as encouraging as they are disturbing. You will start to remember moments that you had hoped would never resurface. This is normal. This is natural.

At this point, you may feel you have just removed an obstacle that has delayed many a successful climb. This is not the time for your ego to rush in and claim any victory. You must first learn to manage your anger before you even consider facing those you once hated. But you do need to start to see that you had help. Your anger has caused many words said in fits of rage to hurt all involved.

Perhaps now you can see you have lost enough, and now is the time to start learning how to use meditation to avoid future loss.

CAMP 2 SHORT-LISTING FEARS

Another new Short-List cognitive tool is needed in order to address the other human basic emotion: fear. This is not a simple matter either, and the idea alone causes fear. To admit fear is seen as admitting weakness, and if you have proven anything, you are not weak. You may be low in confidence, and suffer with indecision, and doubt your ability to get well, but weakness? Never! It is important to know right away that fear is not weakness. It is an emotion that reacts often without logic, and can leave you paralyzed by indecision. Therefore, it's time to take a good, hard look at it and learn how not to live under it.

How do you manage phantom emotions (fears) when you have lived as if they are real for so many years?

First, you list them.

Directions: Get another piece of paper and grab your pen.

You will use the same format as our *Short List* of Angers. Only the questions are slightly different.

Q1: What am I afraid of 2-Day?

Q2: Briefly, why do I have these fears?

Q3: How do my fears make me feel?

Q4: How long have I held these thoughts or feelings?

Q5: Do I like feeling this way?

Q6: Has this fear happened to me? (Is it rational or irrational?)

Now, create a new Short List, a "fears list." You'll find that it will look like the example shown, **Example Q1** Fears, when you are finished.

If you have been afraid to face the question of "What do I fear?" because it might imply that you are weak or somehow unable to face your current conditions, now is the time to show yourself how brave you are.

By identifying your fears, you are half way to letting them go. Ask yourself this:

"What do you not want to happen to you or someone you love?"

Begin your list with this self-commitment: [M] "**I will be honest.**" Now pick up your pen and list all the fears you have right now, today. You may need to look at **Example Q1** Fears to get an idea of what a short list looks like. Then list your fears honestly. Note: *If you have just written your first Short List of Angers, this Short List of Fears will follow that same format. The same tips of writing north and south versus left to right apply.*

Q1: What am I afraid of 2-Day?

Example Q1 Fears:

Of Getting well

Being accepted

*That my mother really
did not love me*

Losing it all again

Of losing my spouse

Of jail

Of having hope

Each person will have different fears. Your fears are going to be very different than your neighbor's. They're all just as important and real. Start by just putting them on paper 2-Day. After a while, you'll find yourself going backwards, and looking over your life, and all the fears you've carried over many years. This weight is enormous. After you list them, continue just as you learned to do in creating your Anger Short List.

Next to each fear, list the reason for this fear. Why did we have it?

Q2: Briefly, Why do I have them?

Example Q2 Fears:	Why (briefly)
Of Getting well	**It never worked before and I am scared of failing again**
Being accepted	**Tired of having to defend myself**
That my mother really did not love me	**It hurts too much, and I loved her so**
Losing it all again	**I can't do it again**
Of losing my spouse	**Everything I touch I lose, and I don't know how to change it**
Of jail	**It sucks there, but it's so scary being out**
Of having hope	**I can't afford another failure. It's too hard**

Listing your fears can be far more painful and difficult than listing your angers. Never discount the possible need for professional therapy if you uncover something that needs more discussion. This Fears List is an excellent tool, but if you're suffering from a mental illness or depression you might want to consider doing this under professional guidance.

Be aware that many people do suffer from clinical depressions in the first stages of getting well. You are not alone. But also keep in mind that depression is a withdrawal symptom of every substance detoxed from your body, referred to as substance abuse mood disorder, and should not be confused with clinical depression.

And do not use this as an excuse to avoid writing your Fears List. Continue on, move on, and learn to climb higher. If you are able to do this, do it now. Don't delay until you feel better mentally. If you need some need extra time to heal after detoxing and before you start your Fears List, seek professional help. It takes an average of two weeks before a person's mind starts to be calm enough to even consider taking any actions while detoxing. A safe place like a professional therapist's office allows you safely to heal your mind and body from years of abuse.

Just as you did in listing the effects of anger, now examine the effects of your fears. Against each fear ask yourself, Did it make me feel insecure? Did it make me feel embarrassed? Did it make me feel sad? Did it make me feel guilty? Beside each fear list what it stopped us from or allowed us to do. Again, avoid short cuts. Do not shortchange your personal state of wellness by letting someone hand you a work sheet with a list of fears for you simply to check off like a laundry list. Your future is at stake; only you can take on this task, and get well.

"Did this fear, make you feel (fill in question with list below)?" If yes, write the feeling it affected beside the person name:

Insecure	Embarrassed
Sad	Guilty
Disconnected	Anxious
Prideful	Jealous
Envious	Obsessed
Lonely	Superior
Inferior	Threatened
Betrayed	Lost
Overwhelmed	Confused

Writing these feelings out allows you to take ownership of them. If you have a fear of poor penmanship or that you cannot spell, that is just another fear. This is not a handwriting contest. Perfectionism is not bad unless it stops you from ever doing anything because you think that if it is not perfect, you won't do it.

As before, you will discard this list almost as soon as you write it. However, write you must, since keeping fears in your mind for years has often clouded your thinking. This is something that Jungians call "psychic poison." This raises its defense by not writing. Where your conscious mind tries to push the problem into your unconscious mind, since facing it openly would seem less than human.

Q3: How do my fears make me feel?

Example Q3 Fears:	Why (briefly)	Makes Me Feel
Of Getting well	*It never worked before and I am scared of failing again*	**Embarrassed, anxious, envious, inferior, threatened, guilty, sad, insecure**
Being accepted	*Tired of having to defend myself*	**Inferior, sad, insecure, embarrassed, anxious, lonely, disconnected**
That my mother really did not love me	*It hurts too much, and I loved her so*	**Sad, envious, insecure, jealous, inferior, insecure**
Losing it all again	*I can't do it again*	**Embarrassed, insecure, anxious, inferior,**
Of losing my spouse or partner	*Everything I touch I lose, and I don't know how to change it*	**Inferior, insecure, anxious, embarrassed, sad, lonely**
Of jail	*It sucks there, but it's so scary being out*	**Angry, sad, envious, insecure, embarrassed**
Of having hope	*I can't afford another failure. It's too hard*	**Hopeless, alone, insecure, embarrassed, sad**

So now you have a nearly completed list, you have listed your fears, and you have looked at how they dominate your life. If you study the example shown in **Example Fears Q3** you can see the effect the feelings it brings up. *How many years has this fear dominated your thinking?* Is it any wonder you are hurt so quickly, when you carry this burden with you daily and when you look at the effects, they affect every area of your daily lives. Fears are crippling: you must learn to live without them.

Now, as you did before when you looked at anger, cover the first three columns and look at the effects of fears in your day. Study them carefully, without the fear that you listed. You can once again shake them up, move them around, and see how they affect all areas of your life. And exactly like anger, they tend to dominate you. And as you learned about anger, you can actually place a time frame on how long these fears have been a daily part of you. See **Example Q4** and **Example Q5** as the guide.

Q4: How long have I held these thoughts or feelings?

Example Q4 Fears:	How long	*Why (briefly)*	Makes Me Feel
Of Getting well	**5 yrs**	*It never worked before and I am scared of failing again*	Embarrassed, anxious, envious, inferior, threatened, guilty, sad, insecure
Being accepted	**21 yrs**	*Tired of having to defend myself*	Inferior, sad, insecure, embarrassed, anxious, lonely, disconnected
That my mother really did not love me	**26 yrs**	*It hurts too much, and I loved her so*	Sad, envious, insecure, jealous, inferior, insecure
Losing it all again	**15 yrs**	*I can't do it again*	Embarrassed, insecure, anxious, inferior,
Of losing my spouse or partner	**5 yrs**	*Everything I touch I lose, and I don't know how to change it*	Inferior, insecure, anxious, embarrassed, sad, lonely
Of jail	**2 yrs**	*It sucks there, but it's so scary being out*	Angry, sad, envious, insecure, embarrassed,
Of having hope	**15 yrs**	*I can't afford another failure. It's too hard*	Hopeless, alone, insecure, embarrassed, sad

Q5: Do I like feeling this way?

Example Q5 Fears:	*Why (briefly)*	Makes Me Feel
		Embarrassed, **anxious**, envious, inferior, threatened, guilty, sad, **insecure**
		Inferior, sad, **insecure**, embarrassed, **anxious**, lonely, disconnected
		Sad, envious, **insecure**, jealous, inferior, **anxious**
Q5 Do I like feeling this way?		**Embarrassed**, insecure, anxious, inferior,
		Inferior, insecure, anxious, **embarrassed**, sad, lonely
		Angry, sad, envious, insecure, **embarrassed**
		Hopeless, lonely, insecure, embarrassed, sad

Once you see how Fears affect you, you can learn to release them. In most cases, the question of *Is it even true?* needs addressing. Have you believed a lie? Often fears, like anger, can span years, and somehow a hidden truth, secret, or lie – if repeated enough – becomes your truth the psychic poison. Then that feeling you believed creates a fear of something that never happened to start with? We have all lived in that state of mind, some of us for our entire lives. Men and women who have substance issues have no market cornered on fears. We simply suffer under them differently than those who did not enter our dark world. Sometimes we compound them with a feeling of "I don't want them to think badly of me." This reinforces the reason to keep the hidden truth, the secret or the lie in full play.

Reviewing the list of how your fears make you feel, you can stop and ask "Is it true?" You are starting to consider whether your fear is rational or irrational?

You have to face your irrational fears, and your rational fears. What is the difference?

A rational fear is when *you know something to be true but act as if it is not*. For example, imagine a person who, while driving, sped and received six speeding tickets in four months. They did not enjoy getting tickets, but continued speeding in spite of their fear of more speeding tickets. A rational fear also can create an irrational fear. This same person could start to feel persecuted. "They're out to get me" is an irrational fear that starts to form. Sometimes this develops to the point of paranoia.

So, rational fear is when you know something to be true, but act (your behaviors) as if it is not. You become desensitized to fears by repeated exposures to them. The fear of driving can be overcome by years of driving.

Irrational fear is *the belief of something to be true, when it is not*. Here's an example: All police are on the lookout for you. A person becomes overly sensitive to fear. A person may refuse to drive, walk near any streets or roads, or ride in a car, since accidents happen.

Another example of irrational fear was the nation's fear of Y2K as the end of times. But the year 2000 came and passed, without all computers coming to a halt.

Fear is the word used to describe an emotional response to a perceived threat or danger. Irrational fear, which has never happened to you personally, takes hold of you and becomes a false reality. It behaves as a ghost, a phantom emotional memory, of an event, which you never experienced but behave as if it had.

So how do you move from your irrational and rational fears to managing them?

First you need to identify your fears by listing them.

You will sort out rational (behavioral fear) and irrational (emotional fear) by using a simple cognitive (thought) filtering question.

Ask yourself: has this fear happened to you? If not, it may be an irrational (emotional) fear. Or if it has happened, that tells us it is a rational (behavioral) fear, like the person who continued to speed, even while scared of getting another ticket.

Q6: Has this fear happened to you? (Is it rational or irrational?)

One simple "fear qualify test" can be in the form of a helper question, repeated three times. *"Is it true, is it true, and, is it true?"*

Q6: Has this fear happened to you? (Is it rational or irrational?)

Example Q6 Fears:	How long	Why (briefly)	Makes Me Feel
Of Getting well (rational or irrational?)	5 yrs	It never worked before and I am scared of failing again	Embarrassed, anxious, envious, inferior, threatened, guilty, sad, insecure
Being accepted (rational or irrational?)	21 yrs	Tired of having to defend myself	Inferior, sad, insecure, embarrassed, anxious, lonely, disconnected
That my mother really did not love me (rational or irrational?)	26 yrs	It hurts too much, and I loved her so	Sad, envious, insecure, jealous, inferior, insecure
Losing it all again (rational or irrational?)	15 yrs	I can't do it again	Embarrassed, insecure, anxious, inferior,
Of losing my spouse or partner (rational or irrational?)	5 yrs	Everything I touch I lose, and I don't know how to change it	Inferior, insecure, anxious, embarrassed, sad, lonely
Of jail (rational or irrational?)	2 yrs	It sucks there, but it's so scary being out	Angry, sad, envious, insecure, embarrassed,
Of having hope (rational or irrational?)	15 yrs	I can't afford another failure. It's too hard	Hopeless, alone, insecure, embarrassed, sad

Now we cover all columns except the first, and look at the fears we have listed shown in **Example 1.6** below.

Just as you did before with your anger list, you use meditation to remove your years of burden, your fears, one by one that you have listed. Learning this, you go forward, then relying on this new tool, in any moment as they crop up in the future. Fear will return, and to the extent you allow it, it will dominate you if you do not treat it immediately as you did with anger.

Example 1.6 Fears:	Why (briefly)	Makes Me Feel
Of Getting well		
Being accepted		
That my mother really did not love me		
Losing it all again		
Of losing my spouse or partner		
Of jail		
Of having hope		

Depending on the fear, use a few simple methods first. Ask yourself, "Is it happening now? Is it real or perceived, and can you do anything about it?"

Then, use the eye movement to unlock it from your conscious mind. The emotion has the effect much like a visual image in your mind, like the behavior of craving.

You have seen that interrupting the fear is similar to interrupting the craving process. Use the interrupter tools we have supplied first. The Stroop chart and the eye movement tool are both effective tools to unfreeze an event.

Now to move to a deeper-seated fear, those you listed to dig them out. As you did with Anger you imagine them, bring them in to your minds, you will imagine letting them go.

Using forgiveness in a different way, you forgive yourself for feeling this way.

Take a moment to feel that fear in the center of your mind.

And in your mind say to that fear, I forgive myself for feeling this way, but you are not real, I forgive you. I release you now. Exhale, breathe, and relax.

This is what it looks like in action, if you take the example Fears 1.6 as the list.

[M] I forgive myself for feeling that I cannot get well, I see myself gaining strength by releasing this old negative image of myself. I give myself the freedom to change.

What does that look like in your blank form?

[M] **I have been afraid of (fill in the blank), I forgive myself for feeling this way, I release this fear, and I give myself the freedom to live free from it.**

By imagining your fears and then seeing them, and then seeing yourself release them, this gives us power to move past irrational fears. This allows you to move past or through the fears in a safe and guided direction without stopping, even when you are afraid to do so. *You do not wait weeks or months to learn this; you start immediately.* You get well as soon as you have a tool to live with the needed knowledge that all people experience fear. You needed a tool to live with them while they occur, and more importantly not under them or driven by them while they occur. Later you will bring in [M] different meditations to help you gain the experience needed to practice this in fullness.

There is a wonderful Koan that asks: "Is it true?" A Koan is a term used in Zen Buddhism that refers to enigmatic or paradoxical questions used by teachers to develop students' intuition and wisdom. As you get well by practice, you will gain in both.

Reference -www.thebuddhistsociety.org/resources/Glossary.html

Recovery 2-Day breaks a lot of old rules and since we get well 2-Day, You want to proceed to the next camp. Before you move to Camp 3, you must first get used to being at a higher elevation. *Remember climbing Mt Everest is not done in a day, but each day we learn something to make us better climbers.* You use meditations to do this. Now and for the next few days you practice this until it starts be a valuable climbing skill. You do not want to climb to a higher elevation until your new tools become familiar and normal. But this is *not* telling you to delay the climb; it means practice this during your climb; do not stop and wait. We have more to learn. The next part is about learning honesty, in combination with your new tools.

A NEW NORMAL

We use the word normal a lot, and now is a good time to look at what normal is. Normal for some reason is often seen as something bad or reserved for someone else. It is quite normal to feel out of place when things start to change rapidly. Just like you might feel during a blizzard that may suddenly happen on Mt Everest.

We have a friend who was instrumental in making Recovery 2-Day™ possible and his story of normal really teaches a great lesson for us all to see.

Our friend's name is Bill T, and he loved his mother dearly. It was the sort of relationship between a son and mother which changed when he married and started his family, many years ago. His relationship with his mother was a loving one, nurtured over their entire life. It was never a burden to have phone calls or visits and many a weekend was spent in their respective homes with only love as their guide. He also worked in the Hospice community and dealt with sickness and death on a daily basis. He helped men, women, and families of all races, religions, and ages deal with the sometimes sudden or long drawn out process of dying.

This was Bill's normal life. And yes, Bill also suffered substance problems during that same period of time.

A few years ago, his mother died, not suddenly, not tragically. She died because her time here expired. This was not seen as a loss in the sense she lived a long and full life, surrounded by love and affection. Her death was a celebration of her life.

Bill's "normal" changed overnight. The person responsible for his birth, and for his years of being mothered, died. A vacuum of sorts was created. Life became abnormal, because life without his mother was not normal. Corporate America sees grieving as a two-week process, normally in something called bereavement, the time it takes to grieve the loss of a loved one. But Bill was not able to fit the two-week model. It was not normal for him to not call or visit his mother. It was abnormal for them all, his entire family felt the void; she was missing at the Sunday table, his community was drastically changed. He had to learn a new "normal."

The new normal was life without his mother's presence in his daily life. And while the tug of his heart was to set a plate for her, it became normal not to. She was loved from afar.

The reason we tell Bill's love story in all its glory is to show you how life works – how it is similar to the very normal life of a person in substance abuse or dependence, who actually grieves the old life even if it was killing him or her, since it was very normal.

To be thrown in a life without substance problems feels abnormal at first, even if it is something you wish with all your might to have. The lesson of Bill is really very close to what happens in your separation from our old life.

It may be killing you, but there is a very strong sense that it is normal. Then to have it removed suddenly is like walking on the moon. The process of having anger and fears managed is completely abnormal as well. Add that sensation to the lost normal and withdrawals of substances, and you are completely lost at first. You feel defenseless, and you are at your most vulnerable state. So many at the stage will say, "well don't go there," don't remove the anger and fears while you are convalescing. The fires that burn you will eventually burn themselves out. But this is not true. Unless we take the actions to get well, nothing will change.

Before we get too worried, a vote of confidence is needed: It is normal to feel abnormal at this early stage.

LIFE LISTS

One of the first lists you created was called a Recovery Stress List, done in your first days in early treatment and then again, later in your treatment plan. It addressed different life situations then. Now, your ideas or concepts of who is important in your daily life and how you behave and how you feel about them as your conditions change, needs a slightly different tool. You have to see where your anxiety-stress comes from if you are to live long and be productive. This is one of the purposes of the next tool we introduce, Life Lists.

Your tools to this point have been orderly, but each piece is practiced by each individual at different levels of effectiveness. The more you practice a tool, the more comfortable you become. You'll become self-motivated. It feels good to see yourself get better. Cognitive, or coping skills are developed by solving problems. Good therapy is about learning how to solve one problem, and then taking that newly learned skill and adapting it to other areas of your life.

This new *Life List* will and should be looked at often, since you live daily in the hectic pace of your own lives. Common sense says it only makes sense that you need to see what, if anything, is causing problems or obstacles that you face each day, and that typically creates stress.

STRESS

Here you consider daily relationships. You are not leaving your spouses or partners off your lists, since you live with them on many levels. So you consider who is in your life, and how you treat them or feel about them. Besides boredom and loneliness, stress will cause many men and women to relapse. Understand by speaking about relapse, we are not suggesting that anyone needs to relapse, but we know that it happens. Nor are we giving it an excuse by discussing it. Most people view relapse as a failure of treatment or a person not taking recovery seriously. This attitude discounts the disease to a willful misconduct attitude that we hope the recovery industry sees as flawed. We also know some people use relapse as a tool, to avoid responsibility or to have their ways, in a deadly game of give and take.

There are those who use relapse as the excuse to abuse others. Years ago a teenager threatened his mother with, "I'm going to drink," if she would not allow him to use the family car. Anyone can see the childishness of this, yet he voluntarily played a deadly game. Here we see who caused the stress: It was self-inflicted. If the mother gave him the car, the child won the day. He learned that threats of relapse tug at others' heart strings. What happens when the mother tires of this game? Does he then have to relapse, because he feels he has to follow-through on the threat? His immaturity is easy to see. He acted as if he was doing her a favor, by not relapsing, but he did not see the destruction caused by the threats he made; that he was setting himself up for another relapse. Obviously, he acted as if relapse was his mother's fault, since his childish wishes were not met.

When you look at your behaviors in your life, you need to address who is in your life, and how you treat them, since all of this will affect your long-term security.

Short-term and long-term treatment plans must have tools to see, address, adapt, and develop skills that address stress. Stress is not solely owned by negative stressors. A birthday party can be as stressful as an electric bill. In the first days of getting well, simply going to the mailbox, if we have one, can be excruciating. Ruined credit, unpaid bills, legal notices or being unemployed are all conditions we face while trying to get well. If there is, a negative that sometimes occurs or results from going to treatment centers, it can be the false sense of security of being in a protected environment for weeks or months. Life continued on in its rapid nonstop pace, while we have been away seeking help. There can be a feeling or hope that everything is okay, as if our worldly problems dissolved when we were off receiving help.

Life Lists will form or show your inner circle, from which you will expand to your day-to-day activities and relationships. Life Lists will bring up anger, fear, security, and love. You will use the same tools Short Lists, learned previously for each area. Short Lists start to adapt with the appropriate tools. Here we start to develop the, "What is bothering me 2-Day," listing skill.

It would or could include these potential stressors:

- Your spouse or partners, boyfriend, girlfriend, etc.
- Children if present or moved out from home.
- Family members, mother, father, grandparents, siblings, extended family - aunts, uncles, cousins, etc.
- Friends, including family members, acquaintances.
- Work relationships, bosses, co-workers, including whom you do business with, such as your power company, water company, anyone who bills you, etc.
- Daily contacts, the clerk at a grocery store to the fast food establishments you sometimes visit.

We center on the most important areas first: Family (if we have them) and careers, (if we have them). List whom you consider the most important, but you are sure to leave someone off the list.

Directions: Take out paper and pen

Make a list of the all the people in your life 2-Day.

ALL LIFE LISTS START WITH THIS QUESTION:
"Who is in my life 2-Day?"

Followed by the four questions (**Q1-4**), to be asked against each name on the list:

Q1: What problems, if any, do I have with this person 2-Day?

Q2: How do I treat them or behave towards them?

Q3: How does my behavior make me feel?

Q4: What values do I practice or wish to practice with them that I would with anyone else?

Life List Q1 Who is in my life 2 Day?

Life List 1
Spouse/Partner
Your family
Their family
Children (if applicable) living with you or not
Employer/boss
Doctors
Drug dealers
Co-worker(s) who you like and who you do not like
Creditors, rent, household bills etc.
Friends who you used/drank with and who you do not use/drink with
Recovery people, who you used/drank with and who you do not use/drink with

Common Sense Recovery

One message often told to men and women who newly arrive at a recovery treatment program is to avoid people, places, and things which involve past drinking or drugging acquaintances. This advice is often given without explanation. Common sense and good judgment is missing in these types of blanket statements. Most people reject this cookie-cutter approach, and most will acknowledge the counsel but hold themselves to a different standard, *your real life*. So what is it that they are trying to say? The intention of these statement means it is a good plan to avoid the places our drugs came from, or streets where it was used or purchased. Old drinking holes, too, should be avoided in those first days. For many, however, this is very unrealistic.

What happens if all drinking took place in your kitchen at home? What happens if the drug supply is your parent's bathroom's medicine cabinet? Or all of your co-workers are smoking pot on lunch breaks? Or your campus is throwing a party and you are the president of the fraternity?

Did we mention our friend Bill is an ordained minister and that each Sunday service he handles wine offered in his church's Eucharist services? Do we tell Bill, "Quit your career of 30 years, to avoid the people, place or thing?" Yes, sadly some people would tell Bill he should walk away from it all. How about the doctors and nurses exposed to narcotics every hour of their daily routine who have spent thousands of dollars on a professional license? Do they walk away, because they suffer with substance problems? What is told to the person who lives with a medicine cabinet full of pain medications used to treat chronic arthritis prescribed by doctors to their parents?

What happens if, for example, your partner, spouse, or parents drink or take drugs? What happens if you have lost your family and now find yourself living back in your parents' home, no matter your age and they drink or smoke a little pot to relax or sell drugs for an income? These are daily real life circumstances we have all faced.

What happens if you started in recovery and returned to work and all your co-workers are going out Friday night to your favorite bar or dance club to listen to your favorite band? Familiar feelings of it not being fair and lost privilege may return. Your emotions beg you to join in the fun. Euphoric recall is dangerous, since it only recalls the fun times, never the consequences.

Now you begin to see why many view this as willful misconduct. Intolerance, misunderstanding, and ignorance believe that once a person receives treatment, all problems are instantly treated. It is very easy to say to a person, "Well you should just move out!" But how can you say that to a teenager? How about telling the doctor to quit his career? It is not that easy if the roles are reversed. Moral judgments are much easier to make when we are not the person being judged.

What happens if you are in a treatment center and the technician or person in the next bed is selling drugs? It happens. What happens if your friend in treatment, which with whom you formed a close bond, relapses? What happens when that new love, relapses? Do you join them?

How is that for reality and stress? The temptation is to lie and to believe that you can just avoid all that.

Relax, exhale, breathe.

Note: Being or feeling alone are valid reasons to go to self-help groups meetings in your first days, if there is no one else who support your efforts to get well. Peer groups or self-help groups are safe, in those first days. We have shown you earlier the obstacles in certain self-help groups; very often they can be as stressful or dangerous as your office friends can be. Never be surprised if a person in recovery asks you to join them in their relapse. Misery loves company.

We wish we could tell you avoid stressful situations, but that that's impossible. Each person is different, and stressors affect all of us differently. Friends found in self-help groups are usually positive relations, but use caution, of course. Trust your judgment. This makes it so difficult for visitors. How would you know who is helpful and when someone is just repeating, room speak the rooms jargon?

A positive relationship list was part of the Recovery Stress List's goal. Since we cannot simply avoid stress, we must have tools to manage the stress. *Life Lists* show us who or what is stressful, and who or what is safe. It will interlink to tools we have introduced.

Short-list the anger and fear, the moment it happens. You will develop new friends, new social outlets, new social skills, and yes, go out with friends to dance clubs or parties, once you learn to manage those conditions. If you feel that it will tempt you, do not go. Here is a simple tip: If you want to enjoy a night out with music and friends, do so with people who know you no longer drink or take drugs. Yes, use common sense. If you are just exiting a treatment center, do not go until you are soundly on your feet. Your substance problem is not a secret to be guarded or kept as a dirty secret. Family and friends, if they are truly on our sides, want the best for you.

You do not have to enter long discussions with co-workers. Avoid that type of discussion, since stereotypes about substance problems still exist. Avoid if you can, using any negative self descriptor labels such as, *addict or alcoholic* to describe yourself. Those labels do not come off and social stigma associated with them is harmful to all. To avoid embarrassment, simply say, "Not tonight, thanks."

One of the most powerful affirmations learned in the first days, during all of those temptations was told to us this way:

[T] *Recovery 2-Day wants the absolute best for you. Sometimes the answer is, No.*

It is better to avoid, bars, and even certain foods in those first days. Pizza, for example may remind you of drinking beer. But we eat pizza today, without any need to drink beer. And yes, it was odd eating it without it at first. Another simple example, we enjoy dances, Mardi Gras balls, weddings, or any social occasion, where substances are always available. These are fun and sometimes mandatory things we attend. You have to manage them, or you will never be or feel free.

The point here is, allow yourself to postpone going to places that at first may tempt you, until you have developed skills to feel comfortable in any and all social conditions. If you go to a place that makes you uncomfortable, leave. This does not mean you can never return. It simply means, not 2-Day. That was the point of telling you that there are days that are not good for climbing. Sometimes it is safer to rest and relax in the security of a place that is not tempting. If you live in a place that is enmeshed in substance problems, go in your room, read the Stroop Chart, or use the eye movement techniques, the simple stop sign is a quick and effective tool, meditate, or visit a safe place until the urge passes. A lot of relapses can be avoided with common sense when and if you feel that you are under attack. With stressors, you need a way to de-compress, so meditation must be developed. The Chapter *Going Solo with Meditation* is covered later. Note: this *Life List* is going to change, often. Your life without substance problems change. You grow into your new normal, which becomes life without a substance problem. It feels awkward at first and then it is completely normal, safe, protective and secure. It's not easy, but you can do it.

The Stress of Change

The stress of change, affects the direction our *Life List* takes. It adapts to the changes in your life. Each question is listed and used in an example, as in previous lists.

What are some simple examples of life's change? Moving, leaving treatment, a new job, the birth of a child, divorce, a new relationship, new relationships do not simply mean a love interest. They can be a new boss, a new co-worker, a new bus driver, returning to home, or returning to work.

Life Lists adapt to your life, as it becomes normal, and then it must adapt when you bring changes into your lives. But that is not the main goal of creating *Life Lists*. It is designed to show you your behaviors and the start of developing your new or different values.

Daily Life List Questions

The four questions (**Q1-4**), are to be asked against each name on the list after the initial question, "**Who is in my life 2-Day?**":

Q1: What problems if any do I have with this person 2-Day?

Q2: How do I treat them or behave towards them?

Q3: How does my behavior, make me feel?

Q4: What values do I practice or wish to practice with them that I would with anyone else?

Life List example Q 1.
What problems do I have with them?

Spouse/Partner

They treat me like a child; they hide their drinking from me; they do not believe me or in me

Children (if applicable) living with you or not

I feel responsible for them, and blame them

Employer/boss
Doctors

I feel like I'm constantly watched since my last relapse;
Scared to tell them I abused that last prescription

Creditors, rent, household bills etc.

I can't answer the phone, or open the mail

Recovery people,

My friend relapsed, and the other stuff sounds crazy, none of this stuff makes sense. My sponsor never answers the phone, or he talks to me like I'm dirt

Life List example Q 2.
How do I treat them or behave around them?

Spouse/Partner	**I isolate, and lie to them, and ignore them**
Children (if applicable) living with you or not	**I yell at them, and avoid them**
Employer/boss Doctors	**I avoid them, and can't look them in the eye** **I lie to them**
Creditors, rent, household bills etc.	**I avoid answering the phone, and lie that it will be better**
Recovery people,	**I just repeat what they want to hear.**

With **Q3**: Once again, we use the list of feelings generated in short-listing:

Insecure	Embarrassed
Sad	Guilty
Disconnected	Anxious
Prideful	Jealous
Envious	Obsessed
Lonely	Superior
Inferior	Threatened
Betrayed	Lost
Overwhelmed	Confused

(Note: each person is different in how they behave. These examples are not meant as absolutes, but are true in that they are real life examples, shown in various people's lists)

Life List example Q 3.
How does my behavior make me feel?

Spouse/Partner	**Dishonest, embarrassed, guilty, sad, disconnected, envious, lonely, inferior, superior, insecure, rejected**
Children (if applicable) living with you or not	**Guilty, sad, threatened, dishonest, sad**
Employer/boss Doctors	**Insecure, embarrassed, inferior, guilty, Embarrassed, guilty, sad**
Creditors, rent, household bills etc.	**Embarrassed, guilty, sad, insecure, inferior,**
Recovery people	**Mad, superior, rejected, disconnected, envious, jealous**

We begin to see how our behaviors do not match our beliefs or our feelings. In fact, our behaviors show us the stress and anxiety that goes are the result of our behaviors towards others, the cognitive dissonance that we face daily, when we compare how we treat them versus how it makes us feel about ourselves.

Before we consider the **Q4** question, we may want an example of some common values:

Love	Empathy	Open Mindedness
Commitment	Trust	Communication
Honesty	Conviction	Mutuality
Devotion	Discipline	Esteem
Integrity	Family	Appreciation
Awareness	Reliability	Equality
Punctuality	Stability	Compassion
Attentiveness	Affection	Loyalty
Kind Words	Friendship	Caring
Warmth	Intimacy	Acceptance
Respect	Partnership	Dependability
Validation	Dignity	Faithfulness

Life List example Q 4.
What values do I practice or need to practice?

Spouse/Partner	**Honesty, trust, equality**
Children (if applicable) living with you or not	**being there, being responsible, giving my time**
Employer/boss Doctors	**Loyalty, trust, integrity honesty**
Creditors, rent, household bills etc.	**stability**
Recovery people,	**Patience, compassion**

This *Life List* also points out if you are to feel better, your behavior needs to change, and explains why you return to the values questions. What values do you want to practice or develop to make your relationships healthier?

Now the final question becomes a plan of action, restoring values in the most important relationships. And as you have learned with other tools, you meditate over each value. Reach out in your mind, to develop this value or practice it, with the person on our list.

A simple example [M] *I need to practice giving time to my children.*

Another realization that happens when you start using this tool is that you find that you may want to talk about these issues that you have unearthed in the process of listing anger and fears or certain behaviors with the people in your life.

Recovery 2-Day™ deals in the here and now, and now is the time to make the next climb, since your load is getting lighter.

CLIMBING TO CAMP 3
FORGIVENESS

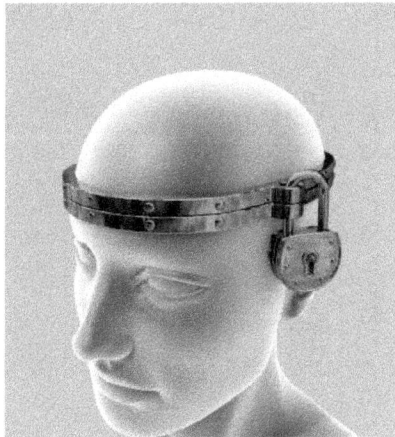

We return to our symbolic climb of Mt. Everest and are about to reach Camp 3, which will prepare us to reach the summit. Our summit will be Forgiveness.

Guilt and Shame

Warning: This next list will create in many the need to talk to someone, in the hope of obtaining a state of forgiveness or freedom. To whom we talk is extremely important, since many have criminal events. Confession is both a legal and religious term.

Most people who come into recovery want to discuss their past, so what needs to be discussed is important. Our experience tells us it is not a long conversation that is needed, but a purging of past events that linger in our memories as guilt and shame. Many hours have been wasted talking about things that do not matter, while trying to decide, Do I want to tell another person this about me? Trust is the issue here. Who you trust is as important as what you are going to entrust them with.

How to construct and properly frame that confidential conversation is critical, since you need to focus on getting well, allowing you to move on in your new normal, life without a substance problem.

If you remember, you created a Regrets List when you first arrived in Recovery 2 Day. If you kept it, you can reuse it here or create a similar list, A Guilt and Shame List. If you did not create a Regrets List, take a piece of paper and pen and before you start, Meditation, think, [T] I need to be honest here. In the beginning, you used the Regrets List to determine if you had an abuse or dependence problem, according to the APA's DSM IV-TR criterion. You also saw that it revealed much more. It was about being honest with yourself about past behaviors towards yourself and others.

If you need an example, it would look similar to this:

Example: I feel ashamed of, and/or, feel guilty about? And for how long?

I feel guilt and shame about this		How long ago did it happen?	
Cussing out a loved one	X Time	Lying to a loved one	X Time
Losing my children	X Time	Being gone	X Time
Losing my job/career	X Time	Having a substance problem	X Time
Going to jail/prison	X Time	Being out of compliance	X Time
Getting caught	X Time	Not being faithful	X Time
Breaking the furniture	X Time	Abusing my spouse/partner	X Time
Letting everyone down	X Time	Letting myself down	X Time
Losing my self-respect	X Time	Having to move back home	X Time
Quitting school	X Time	Driving the kids to school hung-over	X Time
Relapsing	X Time	Not living up to the goals I once had	X Time
Cheating on my partner/spouse	X Time	Having sex with strangers	X Time
Being a dealer		Hustling	
Stealing time		Stealing from family	
Stealing from friends		Stealing from children	

IMPORTANT: Trauma Events such as rape, violence, and incest need to be addressed in professional settings sought through professional counseling

This list creates a structure of the things we want to discuss. We know many hours have been spent reliving, retelling, and re-feeling these events. When we listed How Long in Short Listing angers and fears, often these regrets were associated with the feelings of guilt and shame. Is there one word that can sum up the entire experience of regrets, guilt, and shame?

What did your list reveal to you? Can it all be summed up by one word, Loss? How long have you felt some deep feelings of guilt and shame, causing you to feel disconnected with embarrassment or pride?

We do not associate loss with loser. We see the absence of something, not the winning or losing of a game. Life is not a game to be won or lost. It is the experience of life that all people suffer pain, sorrow, and loss, and on an equal basis we enjoy, happiness, peace, and prosperity. These components of our lives, are subjective. "To each his own," is true, yet we also know, "feelings are not facts." All people experience feelings in different degrees at different times. Some would describe an event as causing them huge amounts of anxiety, while someone else, faced with the exact same problem, shrugs it off as no big deal.

Is there a difference between the feelings of being caught which may produce a certain shame, and confessing what we have done, by an admission of guilt? We may want to discuss lost values. What does it feel like to know better but not do better? Knowing you carry the guilt, and then living with the shame of knowing these feelings, can hang over you like a cloud.

What happens when these events happened fifteen or twenty years ago? While you may carry the guilt or shame, do the other people, if they are alive, even remember it?

In Recovery 2 Day™, when we carry this guilt and shame, where do we go to relieve it from our conscious mind?

What do we know about the men and women arriving in recovery? They carry events that haunt them, often cloaked in silence due to the judgment they fear of others towards the things they have done outside the social standards of their own peer group, environment, or upbringing.

This may sound very confusing so we can simplify it with the most common events discussed in private. The most common shame and guilt we see in the recovery industry revolves around sex. Some events include, trauma, violence, or a substance-induced behavior, that under normal conditions, we would have never entertained. To make a list of these events is impossible, since they are all determined by a person's perception of guilt and shame.

"What would you think of me if I were to tell you this?" The *Regrets List,* or newly created *Guilt and Shame List*, reveals guilt, shame, or both, from doing something, or not doing something. This brings up the years of shame, associated with the loss. It may have been loss of innocence, or a lost value traded for one night, or a series of events from a past spent in a substance problem. To heal this, we climb to Camp 3.

There are two questions that haunt most people: "Will you accept me, if I tell you what I have done?" and, "Will you forgive me, for the things I have done?" The answer most people want to hear is yes. However, the honest answer may not be what you want to hear, which is, some will accept and forgive you, and some will not. There is one type of personality that lacks the consciousness of right, wrong, remorse or empathy, the attributes of a psychopath, avoid this person, they will not help your recovery. **Note**: *This does not mean a psychopath cannot get well, but our methods are not suited to someone that needs years of behavioral training in the absence of conscious, a new set of "right and wrong" rules are needed and Recovery 2 Day is not the one to do that. A trained professional psychiatrist is their best chance at recovery.*

So you are dealing with doubt, mistrust and fear. Fear blocks us from moving forward. Fear sounds like this: "What will you think of me" or "Will you repeat anything I have told you in confidence?" Therefore, while there may be an internal desire to tell someone your past history, the reality of, "Who can I trust" becomes the obstacle. As we have seen, fear and the fear of judgment causes a lack of trust. And many of us have legal issues, so trusting someone with our past introduces all kinds of personal dilemmas.

We must be clear on one subject: there is no such thing as a confidentiality law, which protects or stops a person from repeating what you may tell them *in any self-help recovery system*. Be careful with whom you choose to reveal the intimate details of your life. To be clear, there are only a handful of people that carry this legal privilege, technically called "privileged communication." There are certain ordained sacramental priests or ministers, legally recognized spouse, licensed psychiatrists, licensed therapists, licensed attorneys and licensed doctors that carry this legally recognized privilege. This means if you need to share something and must have a guarantee of confidentiality, these men or women are your safest choices.

Before we go further, and to avoid any misunderstanding, we fully support the sacrament of confession or penance for anyone who believes in it. Some of us have found wonderful relationships with the men and women of religion and offered our problems to these properly ordained people, received absolution, and went on our way. However, having said that, only small percentages of people hold this same belief. *We have many agnostic and atheist friends that see the value of privileged communication without having to convert to a religion or practice.* We only want to make it clear that this option is available, regardless of personal belief. It is safe, and it is free.

On the other hand, we know a majority of men and women enter recovery through inpatient and outpatient rehabilitation centers commonly called treatment centers. These men and women have access to licensed therapists, doctors, and psychologists, covered under this same protection of privileged communications. Common sense tells us that if there is a shame and guilt event, including trauma, these licensed professionals are also the right people to trust, since they are licensed and bound to keep a confidence.

Do you want people's forgiveness, or self-forgiveness? Or a clear conscience? Depending on whom we asked that question, we would of course receive a different answer. Each person is uniquely different, with personal views on this subject. This tool, the Guilt and Shame list, supplies the topic that needs to be discussed.

But we have not met a person who does not want to be forgiven and accepted. We had to find a way to solve the problem of, "Will you accept me and will you forgive me?"

At some point in each person's life, it seems they all want to hear, "I forgive you."

THE DESCENT
SEX AND RELATIONSHIP LISTS

A Warning Must Be Added Here

Warning: *For the person entering this who has experienced a trauma event, such as rape, incest, violence, etc., we urge and support your decision to complete this portion of your recovery program under the care of a licensed professional therapist, psychiatrist, or psychologist. Mental health is exactly what it says--health for our minds. Never be ashamed or guilted away from seeking professional help.*

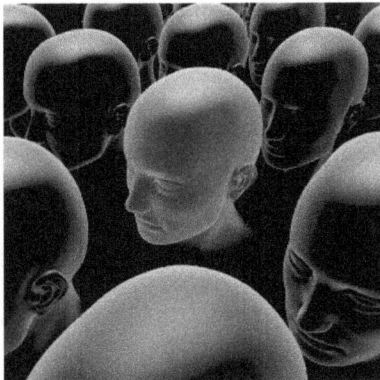

Where we go next in Recovery 2-Day™ will stir as many opinions as there are visitors and members. You need to be warned of certain traps in recovery.

Like the ice crevice on our Mt. Everest, is full recovery too dangerous to even attempt? No. " The Descent" is not meant as a downward spiral; it is coming off the mountain and returning home. This is where your life meets the day-to-day tests of our daily practices, and you are now faced with the reality of life without a substance.

Before we start, let us reassure you that from the listing techniques you have already been shown and practiced, you already have the correct tools to cope with our next subject: security, sex, love, and relationships.. For example, by creating Short Lists of anger or fears, most of the emotional turmoil created by this topic of love and sex came out in those short lists. And if it was not covered there, then it was captured when we created the Guilt and Shame list. This list produced in many the need to have a confidential conversation with someone trustworthy who offered complete confidentiality.

In our experience, the area of sex and relationships is the most often avoided area and the most abused topic in most recovery systems. While the common models ask not to be the judge, when it comes to sex and relationships, it seems everyone is an expert judge. We are not to be judges or judged; however this topic does require self-judgments. Some need to be helped with skills you may have never had but wished to have. The abuses in recovery in this highly personal matter can be seen in anything from movies to comedy shows, treatment centers, self-help groups defined as fellowship's meetings. We need to approach this part of our recovery as part of a mature audience.

This all starts mainly with misunderstanding over words used lightly but highly subjective, such as relationships, love, and sex, since a relationship can involve many things, or the absence of them. Any relationship can be devoid of love, and devoid of sex, and yet to the members of it, be considered as successful. It is completely determined by the eyes of the beholder.

Since we are dealing with the problems involved with a substance problem, we will speak to what we see most commonly in the first days of entering recovery.

It will be beneficial to you by understanding our theory of this word love. It is difficult for anyone suffering from substance problems to tell the difference between the feelings of reward and pleasure. The substance with which we had a problem supplied the feelings of reward pleasure associated with the emotion love. Being separated from either, we experience withdrawals, pain, and suffering. And since this new absence has been self-created, the absence of the reward and pleasure of a substance, there is a sense of self-loss that seeks to fill the imbalance. And most seek or want an immediate solution to the absence. This absence of reward and pleasure, creates a sense of loneliness or loss. This sets up a sequence of events that is predictable. New to recovery, many walk in to a room full of potentials to replace this loss. Yes, many people are attracted at first to the new people they see in rooms called recovery, since they think, They are like me, and we are all in this together. This can create another feeling of this recovery world is my new world now. Let us make the most of it. As though you have moved from the big world, to a small fishbowl and nothing new can enter. This is actually very shortsighted, believing that what we see now, is not going to be different in the near future.

Recovery Sex Rules?

Another rule in some self-help groups in the recovery industry is to refrain from all sexual relations in the first year. This is tied to another rule, which is to avoid making any major decisions in your first year. This second rule is often stated as a form of protection to support the No Sex Rule. This kind of thinking builds steam as it goes, and now has the recovery nickname of The 13th Step. A person is labeled a 13th Stepper if and when they enter a sexual relationship with anyone with less than one year of abstinence. With this blanket statement, a moral judgment is made. It implies that casual sex is rampant among certain individuals in the recovery industry. This derogatory label, The 13th Step, is assigned by people who typically view themselves as morally superior to the persons being labeled as 13th Steppers. Instead of teaching coping skills, avoidance becomes the message.

We, as guides, offer this warning to all women and men who enter rooms which are called recovery in any self-help system, from outpatient to group-step, or non-step recovery industry meetings:

There are men and women who prey on both visitors and members and will seek out an unsuspecting person for sexual gain. Since the rooms are made up of both men and women, we can only advise you to use common sense and be cautious. Some view these places (treatment, meetings, and recovery rooms) as bar's without booze, and predators are there, but this is true of any place where men and women mix. Loneliness drives many to extreme behaviors. Not everyone you meet in meetings is there to get well, and all newly arriving people are at their most vulnerable, making them easy prey.

Common Sense Rules

What happens in a year, and why a year? The answer is people change, but only if they do something to promote that change. For people who wait a year and do nothing besides attend self-help meetings and stop using a substance, zero changes will occur in their relationships, be they sexual or non-sexual. It's just more magical thinking.

We are not recovery police, or your parents, nor do we want to establish any such rules. We do ask you to use the tools before you enter any new relationships, since you will then have a much healthier attitude toward what you do in the privacy of your life. Failed relationships can be very painful, and loneliness may drive you to seek instant gratification. Unhealthy loneliness brings the codependence thinking , best described as *seeking my other half* of hoping that perhaps someone else can fix you and make you feel whole. How can we expect to avoid old behaviors, if we do not inspect our current actions closely, and then if needed, develop new behaviors? Our euphoric recall here more so than other areas, plays games with what really happened, when compared to what we remember happening.

What is the right tool to inspect your relationships? Life Lists are the simple method we find most helpful.

First remember our name is Recovery 2-Day™, not retelling of a life spent in active substance problems. 2-Day means "now."

We are not attempting psychoanalysis, which is finding the root cause of an unconscious mind. Cognitive behavior deals in the now. What is bothering me now in my conscious mind and calls on common sense.

To repeat the Life Listing technique here, is to show you the way it adapts to all conditions.

What are the questions asked after you started the list with **Who is in my life 2-Day** now currently.

Q1: What problems if any do I have with this person 2-Day?

Q2: How do I treat them or behave towards them?

Q3: How does my behavior make me feel?

Q4: What values do I practice or wish to practice with them that I would with anyone else?

Look closely at this **Q1** or question 1 above. Suppose your partner or spouse, or potential partner or spouse is on the list, and they are the only person on the list. It is a relationship list and more importantly, it is NOW, and completely current, since we cannot undo our pasts. And we addressed the past with the Regrets, Shame and Guilt lists so the past remains in the past. However, using the Life Lists, we can create a healthier future for all relations.

Q2 How do I treat them or behave towards them? Then Q2 "Is love present?" and we know that word is subjective. The rest of the questions are easily followed, creating a true self-judgment.

Now suppose a single person is creating this Life List and just walked in feeling very alone.

And the feeling of "I am alone" is pushing them to "fix that."

We look at:

Q1: The problem is myself, feeling alone

Q2: Really starts a self-judgment. How am I going to treat myself?

Q3: How does feeling alone make me feel about myself?

Q4: This becomes the test of self. Will I trade any values to solve my feeling alone?

This tells us, Life Lists really address many areas, including all past or present relations, which include every area of our lives. Common sense allows us to get well in degrees, without the need of years of guilt and shame. Life Lists are a tool that allows us to monitor our values and boundaries.

For those of you seeking more professional help in relationships, consider reading *The Seven Principles For Making Marriages Work*, by John M. Gottman, PH.D. and Nan Silver.

GOING SOLO IN
MEDITATION

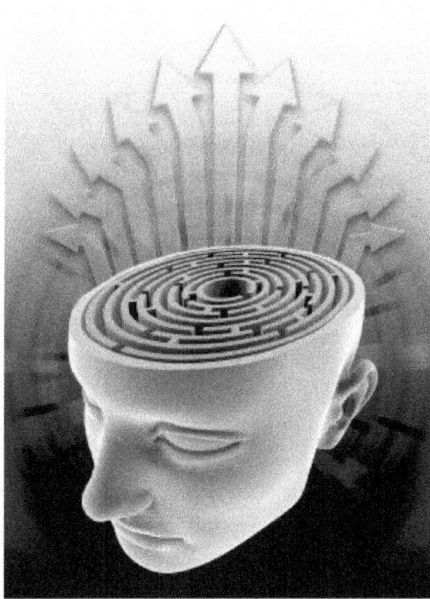

On our daily climb of ups and downs, we face so many obstacles, from boredom to chaos, crisis to peace. One tool rarely mentioned of is how to meditate. In some recovery systems, it is assumed that you know how to meditate effectively. However, at Recovery 2-Day,™ we found most did not, and that is the reason we inserted the practice with each cognitive tool offered. We start with certain times of the day so the practice can flow out into all parts of the day. But for that to happen, you first need a dedicated time, a start and finish time, to enable the practice to develop naturally as you develop your skills.

Each tool shown in this chapter comes with time element instructions of how long to practice it in minutes. Some people will enjoy one method to another. It is not to be understood that each tool must be practiced: the key to Recovery 2 Day™ remains choice and the ability to learn each tool as separate parts or modules and tie them together as needed. However, do practice each of them at least once to gain the experience. How else can you discern which method you prefer? This way, too, you are leaving the door open to try another technique when the time is right.

We have to move past the legacy of dogmatic fundamentalism, sequence-based permission ideologies, that keep people restrained in a belief that degrees of recovery are beyond their reach. Numbered recovery systems, while offering certainty to some, unknowingly, create dogmatic sequence concepts to others. Being out of sequence, produces a long-term negative concept, heard in these words, "I'm not there yet." It creates a recovery class system, of sage and novice, as if meditation is reserved for the elders and not a lesson for the newly arriving. This sage class ego concept, when compared to novice class is always based in lack of time in recovery.

To break this dogma, the tools developed in Recovery 2 Day™ are in a logical sequence, based on the observation of how men and women arrive seeking help. This does not mean a person arriving only minutes ago cannot enjoy the power of meditation before they create a *Short List*, or *Life List*. It could be the tools found in the meditation chapter were the only tools they sought. To repeat our core beliefs, Recovery 2 Day is both a short-terms treatment and a long-term treatment, that choice remains, and is returned to its proper owner, you.

This chapter, while near the end of our book, can be introduced to anyone in the first days or hours of an entrance into recovery. For many meditation has been either a mystery or a routine, hours spent repeating words without any real consideration or thought.

We need techniques that will allow choice, growth, and self protection. We need to develop this practice, to be done at certain times or surrounding events of each day. Our meditation practices must be flexible as if wearing a loose robe, with room to grow. Each evening the old robe comes off, and each morning the new day allows for constant change.

The first technique is called the *Defensive Meditation*. This Defensive Meditation is focused on a particular troublesome event, as opposed to a vague generalization. We meditate and much like a surgeon, perform laser surgery on a specific problem.

Since you have spent the past few weeks listing, you may have found certain areas in your day-to-day life that bother you. The first question, "Do you think you have a problem?" now takes on new meaning.

What bothered me **today**? Keeps your focus on the now. "What is bothering me 2-Day, currently?" Every previously introduced tool has shown you, in some area of your conscious life, what disturbs you and removes you from the peace you seek. Moreover, just how bothered you become disturbs the rest of your day. In this state of mind and emotional distraction, you are prone to say or not say, do or not do something you wished you had or had not said or done - but the event is over, and these thoughts are happening in hindsight. This wishful thinking becomes desire, your internal desire to un-ring an external bell. Yet those moments of regret can attach to you for years, if not decades. We called it the knee-jerk reaction in earlier chapters.

It can happen with a co-worker, your families, your friends, and your own behaviors in split-seconds, with damage that lasts a lifetime in some cases.

We often use the Wal-Mart example since it seems to be a familiar experience. Often we become impatient with lines or crowds and our internal unrest is reflected externally to those people who cross our path. Simply standing in line seems to upset many of us. It happens in traffic, too. It can also happen the moment an alarm wakes us up each morning. We can wake up upset. Since many things bother us, moody would be a good description for many of us.

Little irritations tend to fill our days, and then we take them out emotionally on the people we come in contact with, from that moment forward.

It happens in our jobs and in our homes. Each day presents a different set of circumstances that tends to move us away from our desires to be at peace, as we move quickly from rest to unrest. These daily events really show us how emotionally unattached we can become and how quickly.

Typically this is where a well intentioned person may offer that mysterious suggestion, "You shouldn't do that." But if you are like most of us, while it seems obvious, *how* becomes the natural question. We begin to see that morning, afternoon, or evening meditations have quickly left our memories. The moment our emotions take over, we are separated from our peace.

Therefore, we teach the *Defensive Meditation* now.

We will introduce the Koan, while not a mantra the repetitive nature of it tends to confuse the deeper meaning and often people think it is mantra. A mantra is useful to establish a state of mind, while a Koan is seeking the contemplative state or "thought-meaning" behind the words . Not now, Not now, Not now. These simple words Not now allow us to defer or delay an ill response. It is a simple yet powerful use of meditation.

For example let's consider a simple scenario of going to the store.

We can change the future by protecting ourselves, based on past experiences of being upset, before the event happens. We use the *Defensive Meditation* technique.

We can, before we get in the car and drive to the store simply prepare ourselves, by saying these words: [M] I enjoy peace over being angry.

Of course, we learned that in our short listing of anger and fears. "I forgive myself for feeling this way."

Close your eyes before you enter a stressful situation, bring forth the image of what you believe will cause the stress. Now address it in your mind by saying to yourself: "This will happen, but I will not react to it."

If life were only that simple, we could stop there.

Centering Meditations

"Centering Meditations are an excellent method to open any meeting with or to use at home, at any time. The process has four simple parts to it...It is to be practiced for ten minutes three times a day, or two twenty-minute sessions, to be most effective.

The Guidelines

1. Choose a word as the symbol of your intention to consent to the presence of peace and action within yourself.

2. Sitting comfortably and with eyes closed, settle briefly, and silently introduce the word as the symbol of your consent to the presence of peace and action within yourself.

3. When engaged with your thoughts*, return ever-so-gently to the word.

4. At the end of the meditation period, remain in silence with your eyes closed for a couple of minutes.

"What exactly happens when you meditate like this? Let's examine the process."

1. Choose a word as the symbol of your intention to consent to the presence of peace and action within yourself.

In the first action a word is chosen--as it says, a symbol of our intent. You want a word that best invites peace into your mind's eye (your consciousness).

What words can they be? First, you want to refrain from using more than one word, and try to keep it simple.

What would a word that invited peace look like?

It can be anything…nature, home, peace, love, forgiveness, Mt Everest.

Now, what happens if you have a conflict with a word, like home?

Say for example you are home, and you want to invite peace into your meditation with the same word, home. Can you see how easy it would be for you to imagine your home versus a place of peace? (If your home is like our home, kids, pets, T.V, phones, bills, etc, are distractions).

So, if you can, try a word that does not produce conflicting images. A very easy word often used accepted by all is peace or love.

Remember, use one word if possible, at most two. Less is more. We are seeking a restful state of mind, not a conversation.

2. Sitting comfortably and with eyes closed, settle briefly, and silently introduce the word as the symbol of your consent to peace's presence and action within.

Here we see we are to sit and close our eyes, and then introduce the chosen word as a symbol, inviting peace into our presence and action within.

What is that saying? The closed eyes make sense, the sitting makes sense, but how do we introduce our word?

Image a feather in your mind, and take your chosen word and gently float it down on your mind onto a pillow.

This (closing our eyes) will cause your thoughts to wander.

3. When engaged with your thoughts(*), return ever-so gently to the word.

(*)This is telling you, Your mind *will* wander, and it will do so just as fast as you can close your eyes in the early stages of practice. Do not get upset when this happens. This is normal when you start.

Things we've heard include: "I closed my eyes and in that moment heard my mind speaking to me." "I felt foolish for even trying." "I felt my skin crawl." "I heard my stomach growl." "I wondered if I left my lights on." "I think I look silly doing this, what will someone thing if they walk in and see me?"

This is why we gently float the word on a feather and bring it to rest after each distraction we think or feel.

Questions?

What happens when you mentally looking at the clock, (anxiety)?

Again, close your eyes and return to silence, float your chosen word back to rest without condemning yourself for being a novice.

Do not get upset with yourself, since this practice will require commitment and discipline. It is a skill that we all need to develop, and in time, it will be the most powerful of all your tools.

4. At the end of the meditation period, remain in silence with eyes closed for a couple of minutes.

Here we must set aside time--ten minutes each morning, afternoon, and evening. The time period is important to stay on schedule, since that also helps us to develop a discipline.

Meditation is not about closing your eyes and going to sleep.

It is mental rest. Do not be afraid to explore peace. And if you do fall asleep, do not give up, it is relaxing.

One word of caution: When your mind is quiet, do not disturb its peace or rest. Do not interrupt the stillness.

What happens often is the idea that something needs to happen. Being still is not seen as success, if we expect something to happen.

What happens in our mind's eye when it reaches its stillness? That will depend on the person.

Will peace be with you? Yes. Can you avoid bringing something in to disturb it?

Let us say you have practiced this for weeks. And in that practice, you have found a quiet place mentally in meditation.

But if in that moment of quiet rest, or peace, you repeat your invitational word, you have in essence disturbed your own peace.

The point was to reach a peaceful state. We do not need to disturb it by thinking we need something to think about. But this is what happens often.

The goal is to reach a state of quiet rest in peace or love. No more, no less.

When we end our meditation, then we can move about our day, our mind at rest.

Discipline is the key to all self-awareness. This will need to be done consistently for months in order to become habit.

In other chapters, we mentioned Koan Meditations. Here we intermix and use the guidelines of the Centering Meditation, but instead of selecting our own word, the Koan selects the words for us. Some would call this a mantra. A Koan is not a mantra, it is a mindful statement to show the inadequacy of logical reasoning.

Example Koans:

"I forgive you" (non-traditional Koan)

"Peace be unto you" (non-traditional Koan)

"No" (traditionally the first Koan taught to students) or "What is no"

Note: For more information on Koan, an internet search for Blue Cliff Record offers a compilation of 100 traditional Koans.

THIS PAGE INTENTIONALLY LEFT BLANK FOR NOTES

THIS PAGE INTENTIONALLY LEFT BLANK FOR NOTES

THIS PAGE INTENTIONALLY LEFT BLANK FOR NOTES

THIS PAGE INTENTIONALLY LEFT BLANK FOR NOTES

THIS PAGE INTENTIONALLY LEFT BLANK FOR NOTES

THIS PAGE INTENTIONALLY LEFT BLANK FOR NOTES

THIS PAGE INTENTIONALLY LEFT BLANK FOR NOTES

UNFOCUSED MEDITATION

Relaxed breathing and counting your breaths is a very traditional form of unfocused meditation. Count one breath as you inhale, and one breath as you exhale. To inhale and exhale would be two acts of breathing, count to ten, breathe through your nose to oxygenate your brain and relax. Count until you feel relaxed, and your breathing is not forced or noticed. You could stop there, or add to your practice.

If you are comfortable with counting your breath, do it until you reach the count of ten, and then start over at one. Do this for ten minutes three times a day. For a person first entering meditation, this can be the easiest to practice. When dual thoughts visit you, besides your breathing, simply relax, and gently start your count back over at one and continue. Try not to demean yourself if you feel distracted, simply start your count over.

GUIDED MEDITATION

Guided Meditation is exactly as its name implies: a person directs a group verbally with meditative instructions of either breathing, teaching unfocused meditation, or focused meditation. We have said many times in Recovery 2-Day™ we act as a hallway. Now we use the metaphor of a hallway to help us develop your guided focused meditation sessions. A few things we find helpful while guiding the groups: To avoid noise interruptions, ask the people in your group to turn off their cellular phones. Common sense and courtesy help avoid worldly distractions. A meditation timer if you are alone is useful. Some enjoy the resonance of a bell, allowing them to hear the tone and hear it float into nothingness.

First, relax, and normally people like to sit in a comfortable chair, but a pillow on the floor may be just as comfortable. Close your eyes and listen to the guide. A good guide is patient and speaks with a clear voice. You let them guide you into your safe places and calmly walk you through the meditation.

SAFE PLACE FOCUSED MEDITATION

Safe Place Meditation is one of the most soothing and healing forms of focused meditations. Finding your safe place is about mentally developing your safe place. To create or find your safe place is really very simple. It can be any place your mind considers safe, safe from your past or your present, it does not have to be a place you have been. It can be an image of a place you think would be safe or go for comfort. You will use your safe place to invite people or events into and then release them. For example, if you wanted to forgive someone, you would enter your safe place, rest in your safe place and when ready, bring forth the image of that person and tell him or her, "I forgive you and release you." Moreover, since you are in your safe place, no harm can come to you during this session. While on the topic of forgiveness, it can cover three areas:

- Forgiving someone for harm done to you
- Asking for forgiveness from someone, for the harm you have done
- Forgiving ourselves, for the harm you have done to yourself.

If you are going to practice this forgiveness techniques, you need this safe place to start and return to, safe and protected in your mind. You will walk, float, or travel mentally through your day and open doors to any event past or present that calls for your attention in your mind's eye.

CREATING YOUR SAFE PLACE

Consider now your personal safe place, close your eyes and search out a place you feel the most comfortable being. Peace can be a safe place or your safe place can be a place you invite peace into, so you become at peace. Perhaps this is the meaning of peace be with you.

Later you will create a hallway attached to it with many doors, where you leave and return as often as you like. The doors become symbols of your day, the morning, the afternoon and evening, so you have at least three doors to visit. As you develop, you will build or discover new doors, you will open them and close them, and you will visit them and leave them in the safety of your safe place.

Introducing your safe place and building its hallways

When guided meditations are practiced, guides will direct you to close your eyes and relax, loosen your shoulders, arch your back, breathe in and breathe out normally, then take a deeper breath, in and slowly out, feel your shoulders relax, feel your weight of your legs on your chair, or pillow. Rest in to them. If you can, remember to breathe through your nose. The guide will simply remind you to use the directions of counting your breaths, allowing two or three minutes to settle your mind.

Once more, breathe in, breathe out, and relax.

The guide will help you develop your safe place by asking you to define it, and in your mind's eye, visualize your safe place.

The guide then asks you to breathe in slowly and start to imagine a safe place in your mind, imagine yourself looking around it, and make sure you are comfortable, feel the textures of your safe place, breathe in, breathe out.

The guide asks you to mentally imagine and visualize your safe place. There is nothing mystical or abstract about meditation. Meditation is purely good and very old in design. These techniques can be just as effective while taking a walk.

Your guide may ask if your safe place has a smell, such as a library or porch. Are there sounds such as birds or waves crashing? How does your safe place feel? Is it warm? Can you feel the sun or the glow of a candle or fireplace? This is your safe place, it is completely safe from all worry, free from all fears, and free from all anger. It is peace. This is a wonderful practice to learn if you personally suffered from trauma, or PTSD.

It is a common practice among all self disciplines. Native Americans for thousands of years used sweat lodges for healing and meditation. The sweat was needed to cleanse the body. The safe place was called the medicine place, a place of inner healing. Eastern cultures have been teaching meditation methods for thousands of years.

Now mentally invite peace to your safe place, This is peace, this is peace, and this is peace slowly you repeat to your mind. This is peace. I love my safe place, it is mine.

Breathe in, relax, breathe out, breathe in, breathe out, and relax.

Sit quietly in your safe place, for a minute or two in silence and rest.

Your Guide then asks you to look from your quiet safe place, out into your day.

At this point of resting in your safe place, Your guide can simply take you here to rest. Sitting quietly in your safety, you feel the tensions fall from your day. You could use the directions of the Centering meditation or a Koan of "I forgive you," or "No," whichever you or your guide feels is right for the moment.

Perhaps you have created a *Short List* of anger or *Life Listed* and feel the need or want to meditate on forgiveness. When using the forgiveness meditation, often people like the control of a hallway or door in their minds where they can control who enters with permission. By allowing them to enter your safe place through a door, you can watch them leave the same way. You invite them to visit and you invite them to leave. You can wave goodbye to being angry or afraid.

Your guide could direct you to imagine a hallway. Here imagine a guide speaking as you sit with your eyes closed and being guided this way. The directions can be easily adapted and used in a group or by an individual once he or she gets the idea of a safe place, combined with the hallway and inviting all things to come and go, gaining experience in this technique.

Slowly turn and mentally imagine a hallway attached to your safe place. It has doors, big doors and little doors, funny shaped doors and colorful doors. Relax, breathe in, breathe out, imagine your hand reaching for the first door, and open it slowly.

Invite the person you were angry with into your safe place. Imagine their face and the things that have happened that caused you to be angry. And you tell them that you forgive them by repeating three times, "I forgive you, I forgive you, I forgive you," and "I forgive myself for feeling this way." You can walk them out of your safe place and close the door behind them.

A forgiveness meditation can be said this way or similarly:

For whatever (fill in the blank, example: harm, anger, fear, etc...) you have caused me may I forgive you. It is over, it is over, it is over, and I release you.

Repeat this mentally three times.

Another example is:

For whatever (fill in the blank, example: harm, anger, fear, etc...) I have caused you, may you forgive me. It is over, it is over, it is over, and I release you.

Repeat this three times.

Your last example could be this:

For whatever (fill in the blank, example: harm, anger, fear, etc...) I have cause myself, I forgive myself. It is over, it is over, it is over, and I release you.

NAVIGATING IN YOUR SAFE PLACE

Since a hallway has doors, you symbolically create as many doors as you need. One door could be "my morning," further down the hallway is a door called "my workday," and the last door is "my evening."

The symbolic doors you create can be any person in your life, from your spouse or partner or each and any family member or person you have known in your past or present day-to-day dealings. This practice can safely visit those who have left your life; death and distance can be managed from your safe place.

From your safe place, you have the perfect place to roam around and visit peace, forgiveness, or review your behaviors from morning to now.

The hallway of your safe place is free from worry, free from fears and free from anger.

These practices repeat themselves. This is traditional meditation and the repetitiveness is needed.

I am free, I am free, and I am free.

Now walk out of your hallway and return to your safe place. Breathe in, breathe out, breathe in, breathe out, and now relax in your safe place for two or three minutes.

Feel the textures of your safe place, the warmth, the wind. With all your senses, feel the safety of your safe place. I am at peace, I am at peace, and I am at peace.

Tutorial For Guides

Members have asked for a guided focused meditation to be used loosely, when guiding a group through meditation.

This is written for a guide leading a group. Also, note these same instructions can be easily adapted to individual use. The example will incorporate breathing meditation, then adding the *Safe Place* meditation and forgiveness technique, starting with relaxing and counting breaths:

A bell is used to signal the start, if so desired. Typically, we teach each session in ten-minute intervals. The guides are responsible for timing when the meditation session is over. A bell or a gentle voice is used to start the transition from the meditative state.

Guide: *We start by first releasing the tension of your day.*

Guide: *Close your eyes and exhale, find comfort where you sit, with each breath you exhale, repeat in your mind, 'I release you,' inhale slowly, and while you exhale, mentally say to the tension, 'I release you,' now inhale, and release the tension of the day as you exhale.* (Do this for one minute)

Guide: *Slowly, taking breaths in through your nose, and exhaling through your nose, relax, as you feel your body as it settles into your chair, breathe in, feel the weight of your arms as they rest on your sides, breathe out. Feel the position of your legs and your feet as they rest under you, relax, breathe in, and exhale. Move* *your head by rolling it slowly in a circular motion, release the tension in your neck and shoulders, relax, breathe in, now find a place of comfort for your head to rest in, and feel the weight of your head as it rests on your neck and shoulders. Relax, breathe in, and exhale slowly.*

Guide: *As you feel your body relax, begin to count your breaths, breathing in, is one breath, exhaling is two breaths. As you breathe in, you now begin your mental count, to ten, slowly breathe in, your mental count is one, exhale slowly, your mental count is two. Breathe in, your mental count is three, slowly exhale, your mental count is four,*

Note to guide. The guide walks the group through the first ten count, starting back over at one when the tenth breath is inhaled or exhaled, pausing between breaths to announce the next instruction. The guide could stop here, having introduced basic unfocused meditation. This is the easiest method to start with breathing meditation.

If either *Safe Place* or *Forgiveness Meditation* is going to be the next technique practiced, (do this for two minutes) before the next set of instructions.

Now introduce the *Safe Place Meditation.*

Guide: *Slowly finish your count and inhale and exhale, inhale slowly, and exhale slowly. Now I want you to imagine a safe place, a place that you have been, or have never been but you believe is completely safe to you and always will be. Slowly inhale, and exhale. Bring forth in your mind your safe place. Does the sun shine in your safe place? Are the lights dim? Feel the textures of your safe place. Breathe in slowly. Does your safe place have a familiar smell? Can you feel the temperature of your safe place? Imagine the details of it. Exhale slowly. Are there sounds, birds chirping or the sound of wind blowing between the branches of a forest? Can you sit or stand in your safe place? Feel the touch of it. Is it soft? Relax, breathing in and exhaling. Are there flowers that you can smell, or* *animals you can watch? Is your safe place, floating on a dock seeing the ripples of the water, gently moving to the moons currents?*

Relax, breathe in, exhale. Explore your safe place. Does it have boundaries, does it have walls that feel safe. Are they painted, what colors can you see, is it protective or is it an open space such as beach and ocean, can you taste the salt of the air, with limitless views?

Note to guide. The Guide can describe any concept of a safe place, slowly suggesting, sights, sounds, smells, taste and touch while asking the group to inhale and exhale. When the guide is ready, or finished giving the safe place descriptions, allow the group to rest in their safe places for five minutes.

Guide: *Breathe in, exhale, and relax in your safe place, rest into your safe place repeating mentally, while breathing out, 'this is my safe place', breathing in, 'this is my safe place', breathing out, 'this is my safe place', inhale, 'I am safe here, exhale, I am safe here, inhaling, I am safe here', exhale.*

The Guide can pause or stop here completely, and let the group discover their safe places or move on to the next instruction of building a hallway. *Note to guide.* Most people can easily, compartmentalize their day. By using the symbolism of the hallways they naturally have doors. The doors, then represent different compartments. A door can easily represent a person's morning, afternoon or evening, or a person, place, or thing they wish to inspect or invite.

Caution: Note to guides, do not start out in this next forgiveness meditation if the safe place meditation has not been thoroughly taught or practiced and introduced. Never try to force a person into a meditative situation that they are not prepared to enter. Do not violate the safety of the Safe Place. This practice is highly effective for dealing with past trauma

events. However, we never push a person to any limits which they are not comfortable with or for which they are unprepared.

Caution: Note to participant, do not enter or attempt to enter zones, of memories or doorways that you are not prepared to enter. But since this is done in your safe place, you will remain in full control of who and when each door is opened, if ever, and closed. It is a safe place, and it can be detached as quickly as you imagined it attached.

Guide: *Breathe in, now exhale and slowly imagine a hallway being attached to your safe place. Imagine an attachable and detachable hall, that floats down and attaches to your safe place. Breathe in, exhale slowly, imagine attaching it and detaching it. It only attaches to your safe place when you invite it; it is not a part of your safe place, breathing in and exhaling. Imagine the hallway with doors and windows, breathing in and exhaling. The windows show you, you are still in your safe place, one that you can close the door , or open the door. It can lead nowhere or somewhere; each door can attach to anything you want it to attach. Imagine a safe door, a door that if you open it, opens a memory of joy and laughter. Breathe in and exhale, you can imagine any time or any place you have been or want to visit. Inhale, slowly, imagine you have climbed Mt Everest, imagine the cold, the bright light reflecting off the snow, imagine the view, imagine the feelings of reaching the top of the world, breathe in slowly, exhale, rest.*

Guide: *Imagine a door called your morning breathe in, and exhaling, now imagine yourself walking toward the door called morning. If you open it, it will allow you to revisit your morning, you can revisit any part of your day, by attaching and detaching doors in your hall.*

Guide: *Now imagine a door that protects you from a person, a person who has perhaps harmed you. Breathing in, and exhaling, imagine walking towards the door. When ready, slowly reach for the doorknob. Is the door locked? If so, you have the key to open it; if you are not ready to open it, relax, breathe in, and walk away from the door. Detach the hallway and return to your safe place, relax, breathe in, exhale.*

Guide: *Now imagine you are ready to open the door, breathing in, you unlock the door, and invite the person into your hallway, imagine their face and features, relax, exhale, breathe in, imagine the harms they have done and the reason you want to talk to them. Breathing in and exhale you can say 'I forgive you for the harm you have caused me, and now I release you.' Now you ask them to leave through the same door in which they came and you watch them leave your hallway. Relax, breathe in and exhale, slowly close the door behind them. You are free of them, and you detach your hallway, and return to your safe place.*

Note to guides: Do this for two minutes, allowing the last minute to simply relax if a ten minute session is used.

Guide: *Gently and when ready, open your eyes slowly, breathe in, exhale one last time, leaving the stress of the day as you exhale.*

Note to guides and participants: The same methods all done in the safety of your safe place can be used to feel forgiveness by slightly altering the words spoken when the door was opened.

Example: You can say something like this, *"I ask you to forgive me for the harms that I have caused you."*

Self-Forgiveness can be approached in the same way again by slightly altering the wording in your hallway; you can hang a mirror on the wall of your hallway and speak to your reflections.

"I forgive you"

Peace be with you.

GOING SOLO - DAY LISTING

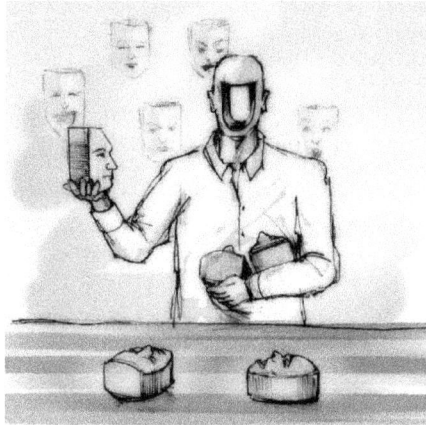

The last tool in Recovery 2 Day™ is called *Day Listing*. It is the culmination of all the tools developed and experienced that have helped you develop your new normal. *Short Listing* anger and fear taught you to manage anger and fear. *Life Lists*, taught you a value system to practice with the people in your life. *Day Listing is* typically used after full remission, since the first months of recovery are so busy establishing your new normal. Your new normal established a baseline of staying quit or a basic level of recovery for you to judge your own success. This basic level of recovery has to be defined so you by using the tools can achieve your initial goal. The question of

"Do you want to quit" answered by "yes" was the baseline for you and those that follow you, who seeks help with a substance problem. If you quit, and that was what you sought, you have achieved your goal.

The final question of recovery is: "Do I want more than just quitting the substance problem I had when I entered recovery?" In addition, honestly, if you achieved that goal, you can call that success. Being substance free is obviously healthier than being substance dependent.

The common sense qualifier to the question "Do I want more than just quitting?" should be, "Did all my problems clear up when I quit?" Moreover, we must allow you to address that question honestly. If you quit and say, *"That is enough,"* then we must respect your personal decision.

Our original question to you, was "Do you think you have a problem," followed by "Do you want to do anything about it?" You then chose, based on your beliefs, to use the tools of the North Pass, the combination of cognitive lists taking gaining insight with meditations. Recovery 2 Day™ then took you through a series of tools that you learned by experience and now practice. Each tool was developed to allow you to live substance free, moving you from a once normal substance filled life, into your new normal. We defined your new normal as life without a substance problem. The question, "Do you want to quit?" was asked, and now you must face or decide for yourself, "Am I done?" "Can I remain quit?" and "Wasn't that what I came for?" Another decision was, "Do I want or need a support system while I firmly establish my new normal?" Some will want the support of a self-help group, while others will not. Each person must decide for himself or herself what is best for a long-term treatment plan.

Most good treatment will establish a goal for each client. Treatment should clearly define its objective that allows for a clear start and a clear end. "What did you come here for?" The end to all therapy sessions is accomplishing the original goal. One question that remains is when do we recover from recovery? Some say never but is that simply fear of being well speaking, and again that is subjective. What is needed is the freedom to come, stay and leave. This allows for each person to produce measurable results. If you came into recovery to quit a substance, have you succeeded? The medical community established this criterion: "Full remission" is considered being substance free for twelve or more months. "Partial full remission" is one month to eleven months, when a person remains substance free during that same time period but has not passed the twelve-month mark. "In partial remission" refers to a person who lapsed during that same period. Recovery 2 Day™ made one promise to you, We get well in degrees. In the harms reduction therapy models, reducing episodes and gaining time between episodes is considered success, that remains to be seen.

We can easily see this in the symbolism of climbing Mt Everest. Some reached the top and returned home. Some are still trying, and some did not. If you have climbed this far, is it time to stop, and this is not an egotistical stance, you can achieve whatever level of happiness, you desire with the proper tools that will allow you to cope with stress of life, without having to return for a substance solution.

On the other hand, a person who asked for more, wants more to enrich his or her new normal.

What you need to establish is change. How do you acclimate to it and once acclimated, how do you notice the little things you typically ignore, which cause you the most problems.

Most people have a question they ask of themselves, "Who am I?" especially when their identity has been almost abolished or defined by a substance problem for many years. It makes perfect sense that if you are now substance free an identity crisis is felt. A natural vacuum, the loss of the substance problem, creates an absence in your identity that needs to be filled. "The emperor has no clothes." This means the emperor cannot see the problem. Therefore, in order for you to see the problem you must establish a tool that collects data about your day-to-day life. A tool that is easy to use, over a certain time period that paints an image of *Who am I,* it should reveal both your weak areas and your strong suites. *Day Listing* will offer you a comparison of then and now. If you do not track your behavior, how would you ever establish a natural desire to change, learn and know where you should focus your attention?

If you asked for more, you need to define what area of your life are you seeking more of? It goes back to the origin of good treatment; I want it all is an immature attitude, since we can have it all only if we address it by its parts. You would need to establish a start and end, that in time, addressed it all. So your personal goals can be set and achieved. *Day Listing* will collect the needed information that will allow you to have more.

If you have seen a children's puzzle game, called connect the dots, you know that children learn by connecting the numbers or alphabet, and once it is done, an image is revealed. *Day Listing* is similar in the collection of dots (days). You will then compare the previous days, creating a true self-image.

Day Listing is going to be done as its name implies, daily. It logically needs to be done in the evening since it captures the entire day's events. It needs to be done over a six to eight week period of time so that you accumulate information about your true self. It requires you to suspend self-judgment, until the end of the data collection period of six to eight weeks.

Day Listing collects data by asking four simple questions:

Q1: What bothered me 2-Day?
Q2: How did this affect me 2-Day?
Q3: What was good about 2-Day?
Q4: What values did I practice 2-Day?

The directions for starting Day Listing are as follows:

Mark your calendar with a start day and end day. This keeps track of your commitment to gather the needed information. Decide before hand, Am I going to do this for six weeks or eight? (The more data you collect is obviously beneficial.)

You will need a notebook with enough paper to cover forty-two to fifty-six days.

Each day gets its own page. If you miss a day, leave that day blank. Extend the collection period for another week to make up for the missed information.

Date the page, and title it Day List Monday, Tuesday, Wednesday etc, each day of the week.

Then answer the questions Q1 to Q4 each day for the time, you have committed.

This gives you empirical data, where a comparison can be seen and actually measured.

When you are finished with the six or eight weeks, you will compare each current Monday to the previous Monday or current Tuesdays to past Tuesday's etc.

Then you can prioritize where you should focus the most energy, home, family, work, etc.

Common sense tells us you will have nothing to compare until it is done for at least two weeks. However, you will not see behavioral patterns until you collect enough personal data, which requires at least six to eight weeks. The reason to avoid mental listing, is also obvious: your mind tend to minimize most of the events that bother you. Writing down what bothered you 2 Day shows you that problems happen daily. However, you tend to adapt to the problem, rather than seeing if you can actually do something about it. We know this is true from the amount of time you listed when we asked the questions in *Short listing,* How long, and Do you like feeling this way. Most people carried those feelings for many years.

After you have collected the weeks of information, compare each Monday to the previous Mondays that you have collected. *Is there a recurrent event?* Do you do something each Monday that upsets you or bothers you? On the other hand, is there a person you come in contact with daily or weekly that always seems to upset you and makes your "what bothered me 2 day" list continuously?

By *Day Listing,* we see the patterns of our behaviors. By connecting each previous day, we connect the dots. We draw a clear image of *Who am I?*

Once this is done, you can then discern which is more important to address? Let us look at a mother with small children and diagram a few scenarios of her days.

Let us say that each Wednesday, she has a task that must be performed that causes her to have anxiety. She *Day Listened,* and answered Q1 with *"I had to go to the grocery store."* The Q2 question was, *"I feel sick each time I think about money,"* and its "grocery shopping." It raised self-esteem issues, possibly of, *"Do I have enough money to buy groceries, there are so many past due bills to pay, and do I tell my family we don't have enough money to do the things we used to do?"* Q3 Was answered with *"at least we have food to eat."* Q4 Was answered with *"I went to the store even when I did not want to."*

What happens when this same person goes to work late, and a co-worker bothers her, since the co-worker goes out of his way to show the boss, "she's late again," and each day of the week, she feels angry with the co-worker. This pattern is common and most people ignore this, and adapt to being upset each day with the co-worker, until it is normal to feel upset. *"It's just part of the job. I hate that busybody, and my boss knows my kid's situation."*

Now let us extend this further. Our mother has small children and takes them to school each day, and since they are small, they tend to run late. This causes her to be late for work, and each traffic light seems to turn red on the way. Frustrated each day when she sees her children making her late, she yells at the children. It becomes normal to yell at the kids.

So what is the point of collecting this data?

First, we would see that running late perhaps is the cause, by simply collecting the data. However, collecting the data does not necessarily mean she changed the alarm clock. It may show her that she is constantly late. Some people are not attuned to self-examination or self-assessment which makes seeing the image of self more difficult. Even writing it down may not produce any new news.

Does that pattern of behavior set up the rest of the week? Perhaps we can use it to change our futures.

What would be the obvious correction if we were to offer any advice? We know that anger is present; we know fear is present and we know that fictitious person's security is threatened. If she continues to be late, there is the fear of losing her job.

First, we are not going to offer advice. The use of the tool was for the person *Day Listing* in order to see herself, honestly, for her to decide. What is more important is addressed in the Q4 question.

Q4, What values did I practice? What values can I practice?

For example, maybe she saw that yelling at the kids is not what she wanted for her children. However, did she tie being late to the yelling? Children can be handful at any age. Would she see being late, was her normal, that to be late was or had become just the way it was, and she had adapted to the discomfort it brought? Would she realize that to get up earlier would solve most of the problems? Would she ever make the connection if she never compared each morning to the previous mornings.

What happens if she sees that each time she visited the grocery store, she became anxious about money? Has she learned to defensively meditate? Has she not learned that being honest creates personal freedom? That she can have an honest conversation such as We don't have the money for name brand kids clothes, but we do have the money to eat.

To insert a non-fiction event, a man used *Day Listing* that had written many hot checks while in his last days of substance problems. Hot Checks means not having the funds in the bank to cover the amounts to which they were written.

Each day he *Day Listed*, he wrote what bothered him, he listed he was afraid of being arrested for having hot checks floating about in his community. After listing this for a few weeks, he finally saw that this really bothered him. While this sounds obvious to anyone that has never had a hot check, it was something he had adapted to. It was part of his accepted problems that came with his substance problem. Then, one day he saw that this bothered him to the degree that he went and paid off the bad checks. Would he have done this had he not *Day Listed?* We cannot say, but we can say he decided it was time to address this, and he did it as a result of listing it daily. It bothered him to the point of doing something about it. His values changed by gathering enough data about himself to see how to fix it.

He was not told to fix it. He learned the value himself since he could not deny what he listed about himself. The ***who am*** I was clear: I am a guy that has some hot checks that need to be addressed. This self-correction allowed for his self-esteem to be raised by self-awareness, seen by *Day Listing*. He listed it for weeks, he was not sure of any legal consequences that he may face. But he needed to clear this up, since he saw his rational fears kept him a prisoner.

The simplicity of *Day Listing* is what it reveals. ***Who am*** *I* can be defined by seeing each day on paper, then collecting enough information about ourselves to see how we react in our daily lives.

Once we have that data, we can meditate over each item we feel is most important, we can discuss it with friends and guides, to learn how they handle life's struggles. In addition, we pick and prioritize which items are more important: Family or work, friends, and the day-to-day life of change.

Day Listing once initially practiced, can be done daily and the self image remains clear. It will reveal each area that we feel needs our attention. This was the purpose of learning Cognitive skills.

The sense of mastery from solving one problem frequently inspires the patient to approach and solve other problems that he has long avoided Aaron T. Beck M.D.

GOING SOLO - BE THE GUIDE

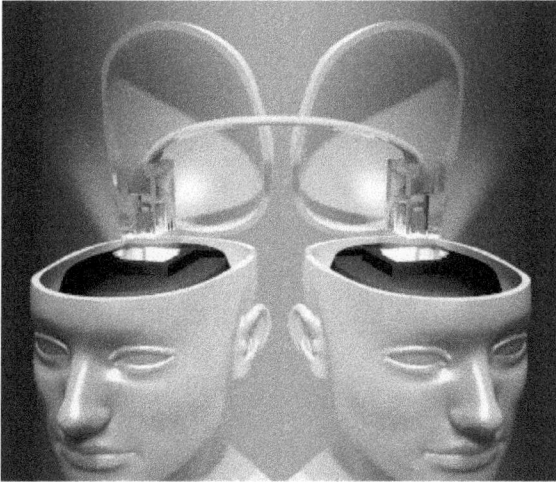

When we entered the climb to recovery we all needed help. We used a guide, this book, and perhaps a friend who had gone before us. We learned that a guide is simply a guide, not a life support system. We learned that having many guides is helpful, since no one person has all the answers. Guides come in all sizes and shapes, doctors, therapists, psychologists, psychiatrists, white-collar professionals, blue-collar professionals, moms, dads, men, women, attorneys, clergy, and average laypersons.

The Guides of Recovery 2-Day™ are the laypersons, even if the visitor is a medical professional, therapist, psychologist, psychiatrist, attorney or clergy. They are off the clock when they come to us seeking help for a substance problem.

The only requirement to become a guide is experience and willingness. It is not the time you put into it, nor the number of meetings you have attended. We're often tempted to try to make a person avoid the same mistakes we have perhaps made. But the best guides offer tools that help people before or after mistakes are made, because mistakes *are* going to be made. By allowing a person to develop his or her own skills, we are enabling them to be able to stand on their own. The feeling of "I wish I had known then what I know now" is universal. Some of us may devalue ourselves and believe we have wasted our lives, and sink into guilt and shame. But this same feeling was why we sought help and eventually got well. This is what made our past experiences so crucial – because it strengthened our desire to not repeat it.

Experience means that a person who learned the skill of short-listing this morning could teach a visitor that same afternoon what he or she has learned. This also means if a person has never short-listed, they should. They need to be honest with a visitor and tell them that they have not done that yet. Our guides tell them the truth, out of their own experience.

We have repeatedly advised them to seek professional help, in all cases of mental disorders that co-exist in many of the men and women who have problems with substance abuse and dependence. Recovery 2-Day™ is a short-term and long-term treatment plan. It is designed for the individual to practice and to get well with, and it works in parallel with those who need professional medical treatment with problems other than substance problems. It is not intended to replace or derail them.

It is designed as a hallway, of sorts. By using our methods and techniques, our visitors and members learn to enter any room comfortably, whether it is a legacy 12-step meeting or a newly created Recovery 2-Day™ meeting. Our techniques allow a person to get well under any conditions. Our members can teach and learn anywhere.

Our philosophy is not based on going to meetings, but in developing skills that allow us to enjoy more family time and actively reenter society instead of avoiding it. We see meetings as an early stage of recovery, not evidence of it. Meetings are important social outlets where we can enjoy each other's company, drink some coffee, and relax. Fully understanding why we attend them, our guides meet new visitors at meetings, and we regard them as a short-term staging area, not a long-term treatment plan.

As laypersons, we cannot treat or pretend we have all the answers.

We need to discuss a term the first generation of self-help groups use called sponsor. Many of our visitors and members visit these legacy rooms on a regular basis. Sadly, over the past few decades the concept of the sponsor has evolved in to a human crutch, or Maslow's nail.

If the only tool you have is a hammer, you tend to see every problem as a nail. ~Abraham Maslow

When problems arise, the most common reply in meetings has become, "Ask your sponsor." The sponsor is the sage to the novice. The novice is told to rely on the sponsor's judgment. In many ideologies, or recovery systems, this transference is demanded as a part of recovery. Terminology is hired and fired used in this fashion: "I hired a sponsor" or "my sponsor fired me." And by having one, we're designated as being a good member. The logic of transference to a superior archetype is based on the assumption that if you qualify for treatment, you are living evidence of *poor decision making*. Using that subjective logic, all members require a person to approve all future life decisions. If substance problems were purely a moral issue, this could be the case, but science has proven dependence is a disease (neurotransmitter dysregulation). This lack of knowledge directly implies that having a substance problem reveals a member's lack of judgment and his or her inability to make proper decisions. Proving it needs to be given to a more developed human that would perform the task for them.

This transference concept is abused to the degree that men and women are being told to call their sponsor to seek permission to use the bathroom. Dating and marriage partners are selected, approved or disapproved. Sometimes a sponsor is even in charge of allowing a person to date. One member of Recovery 2-Day™ was fired by his sponsor and excommunicated from a group because he decided to divorce his wife. He was told that it was not God's will. Members of this legacy are told when a person is allowed to work, sleep, eat and which meetings to attend, and if they are even allowed to speak in them. Many groups have time barriers for when they are allowed to talk (share) and chair meetings. These are just some of the rules that sponsors enforce. It has become a domination system, built over time and egos.

People's medications are reviewed by these sponsors, financial affairs, legal advice, and child rearing all fall into the realm of "my sponsor said." There are men and women so paralyzed in this culture that they will not move without permission. And if they moved away from the sponsor's power, and relapse, they blame it on being absent from the power of their old sponsor. If a person does not have a sponsor and relapses then the lack of sponsorship is in part the reason given. They didn't have a sponsor is given as the reason they drank or drugged. This system is severely broken, but the damage it creates breaks more. This is all flown under the flag of one simple yet extremely dangerous statement: "It worked for me."

Actually, there is one type of personality disorder which does benefit from this militant behavioral punishment philosophy: the psychopath. A psychopath is someone who demonstrates severe anti-social behavior. These types need rigid rules to keep them from prison or abusing others and themselves.

This is the main reason for Recovery 2-Day™ being completely divorced from this methodology and philosophy. We do not use punishment or threats to help you get well. We teach techniques and methods that are healthy and devoid of this taskmaster hire-fire punishment mentality.

Here at Recovery 2-Day™ our guides are not replacements for therapists, professionals, or men and women of religion. We are laypersons. What is a layperson? A layperson is somebody who is not an expert in a specific area, or a non-ordained person. We have experience – experience with Recovery 2-Day™ and life experience.

This means our guides are not going to run your life. We developed tools that help others enjoy life free from substance. We do not take prisoners, nor are we adopting our visitors for life memberships. We do not want or expect anyone feeling indebted to any one or multiple persons or guides. If you want to give thanks, thank God, or your parents, or the universe - that you are alive.

People have become afraid to have an "I know" attitude, since in the legacy model it was seen as not being humble. The word 'humble' is often misunderstood, and used as a battering ram for control. If you want a textbook definition of humility, ours is "know who you are." Or Popeye's "I yam what I yam." Or the single word "be." Be you. Defined in Recovery 2-Day™ as self awareness, this is the highest level of Maslow's *Hierarchy of Needs*.

Another important message to any and all visitors to Recovery 2-Day™ is that some people make very bad guides. No matter how skilled they are in other areas of their lives, some are simply not cut out to do this.

Our methods are experiential, not to be quoted in meetings, but shown in meetings. In other words, we try to say "I do this" rather than "I think this." Experience is the key here, not key chains tracking time or self-inflating egos needing titles. *Friend is a healthy title to earn, so be one.*

Since we mentioned meetings, we will also tell you what a meeting of Recovery 2-Day™ is: a meeting where methods are taught by the men and women who practice them. Our meeting teaches our methods and techniques.

Each meeting starts with at least one technique or tool taught or practiced. Since they take only minutes to teach, coffee, donuts and a notepad, pen or pencil are predictable requirements in each meeting. We do not collect money since our meeting places are free. We have no corporate offices to support.

What is a good guide? Or how do you become a guide?

First read this book, and do what it asked you to do. Then be prepared for the visitor to ask you, Have you short-listed angers and fears? Have you gone to the proper authority (confession), and spoken privately, and been freed from your past? Have you Life Listed? Have you practiced the Defensive prayer or Defensive meditations and seen any results? Have you Day-Listed, for weeks and months? Do you use the Centering Prayer in or centering meditation or the Monk's Ladder? Can you show me a Koan? Can you answer these questions with a confident "Yes." If so, you can be a guide.

And where or how would a visitor know to ask these questions? A good guide will ask them to read this book to see if they agree with our methods and techniques. Since they do not have your experience with Recovery 2-Day™, they need to learn about it first. After they have read this book, they will have questions that only an experienced person can answer truthfully. "Yes, I have" or "No, I have not" are good answers. "I don't know" or "I have done that" are good answers.

Will you be a good guide? We cannot say.

How do you find a person who needs Recovery 2-Day™? Men and women suffering from substance abuse and dependence show up in hospitals, treatment centers, and self-help groups hourly. Walk up to a man or woman and ask them four simple questions:

Do you think you have a problem with either drugs or alcohol? **(Substance abuse or dependence)**

If they say yes

Ask them if they want to do anything about it.

If they do not, do not press them, leave them alone. Always remember, 25% of all men and women who have a substance problem, do not want help with it. It is never our job to try to convince someone they have a problem.

If they say yes, ask them if they want to get well.

You have two choices in that moment, and understand this moment may not come again. When a man or woman comes for help, they may change their minds right in front of you. The worst mistake you can make here is to tell them, Keep coming back, because this may be the only time they come seeking help.

If they respond, Yes, I want to get well, ask them if they want to start right now, 2-Day.

Remember, our name is what we do: 2-Day means now.

Now, understanding comes into action. Are they craving? Or are they jittery? Our experience helps us notice the stage they're in.

Do you show them the Stroop Chart? Yes, that is a good idea. "Let me show you something that may help" is a good first approach. You do not have to understand brain memory functionality to show someone the Stroop Chart. It works for interrupting craving. Just know how to show it to them: Read it, and then read out the ink color.

Then ask them, did your craving subside? Cool, huh? Speak in everyday language, not technically. Get him or her a cup of coffee, or a soda, or water. Sit down and relax, talk to him or her, find out what brings them here. Try to remember how you felt when you came looking for help, scared, ashamed, alone, and it felt impossible. You could be the first person who offers hope and the idea that they are not powerless or unmanageable. We get well by learning tools that empower us and then managing our emotions and feelings. Just one simple question can cut through all.

If you see them craving, try offering the eye movement tool. It is really easy to remember and you may not have your book with you containing the Stroop Chart. So teach them the eye movement to interrupt craving.

You can ask them: Do you have any regrets with alcohol or drugs? Then listen to their response. Let them talk. They will tell you parts of their story. This takes time. You can interject the question: "Do you want to quit?" and "Do you want to get well?" at any time it seems naturally to do so in this conversation. Experience tells us people come looking for help, but they are afraid of the idea of life without drugs or alcohol. Experience knows trust, honesty, and hope are needed in those first hours.

Do not be afraid to take them through the recovery process right then. Show them how you did it. Take out the book if you need a quick reminder. Grab some paper and pen and guide them. Jokingly, you can tell them of the high tech tools we use: a pen and paper. The more you do this, the better guide you become. Practice, practice, practice. Just like all of our other tools, it takes practice. Remember we start getting well as soon as we start. So if they want to start now, help them with it. Do not delay.

Be reminded when someone seeks help, they come with their lives in flames. Do you send them home still on fire, or do you help them extinguish the flames? Some will leave on fire, some will leave in full knowledge they can get well. But they will all leave on fire if you never stop to show them how to put their flames out.

Remember we never use labels. Explain to them why not and how negative it is to them.

If he or she wants to think it over, that's fine. Let them. Tell them how to find the book, and ask them to read it. They may decide to do it without you. However, you have helped, since they did not know about getting well before you had your talk with them.

Tell them they will get well in degrees, and then ask them again: "Do you want to get well?"

Since we have different tools for the agnostic or atheist, you can ask them if they believe in God or not, and if so, what do they believe in. Explain to them that we are not a religion or cult. Recovery 2-Day™ combines cognitive techniques with spiritual techniques. We have no problems with people who belong to any sect-faith tradition. This is important, just as it is also important that they know we won't gossip, we won't repeat their stories, we are safe recipients of their stories.

Ask if you can call them. Do not give them your number and expect them to call you. **You call them**. This old ego of they must call you is simply that, pure ego. If we are to help, be helpful, not dictatorial. If you call and they have changed their minds, which happens all the time, do not worry, toss the number, it did no harm to try. We do not chase after people to get well; there are over twenty million candidates. Help those you can, twenty-five percent do not want help, leaving fifteen million who do. The largest legacy self-help group has 1.2 million members, leaving fourteen million helpless. It is hard to avoid taking it personally. It is not personal or a contest of who is a better guide. Remember, personalities are different. They may hear the exact same thing from someone else and act as if it were the first time they have heard it. We are here to help, not to compete for trophies.

If they are glad you called, ask them if you can help them. Do not give money; do not be taken for rides. Use common sense: if a man or woman wants help, they know you are sincere. They will appreciate a kind word and being encouraged. Do not berate them; they have had enough of that for too long. *Remember if you break it, you have to fix it.*

How do we respond to a person who is searching for something, and unsure of Recovery 2-Day™?

Hand them your copy of this book, or buy one for them, or tell them how to get it. Recovery 2-Day™ makes every effort to be as available as possible.

Encourage them to read it. Give them a few days and call them. Then offer them help if they want it. They will help themselves and there is no better feeling in the world than getting well, especially when they are the ones doing it. Do not be a crutch, do not be a lap dog. Be honest, compassionate, and caring.

Be a friend, not an adversary. If they want to argue, walk away, since you will only upset them and yourself. Life is too short.

If they want to get well, you can teach them the tools we use. That is being the best guide. Then set them on their way. We do not expect them to call us, thank us, or pay us. We do this for fun and for free. Yes, it takes a lot of patience to be a good guide, which is why there are so few of us. Not everyone is able to be one.

What can you do to help when you find someone that is actively using a substance, and they want to quit? Find out the closest detox to you and treatment facilities. Never try to detox a person in your home unless you are insured, and a licensed medical practitioner. A medical professional needs to be involved, since a life may be at stake.

Contact their family, and you can help in the arrangements as long as you are comfortable with the inpatient process. Withdrawals can be serious, life-threatening events. Make sure the family or your new friend understands detox is not treatment. Treatment can only begin after their bodies have been separated from the substance they abused or became dependent upon.

It is good to find out names and numbers of local hospitals that treat active addiction and their procedures to see a new patient. Once a person comes out from treatment or detox, be there to help them. Remember if you take on these responsibilities, you are responsible for helping them. Not to run their life, but to help them in those first days when they start to feel human again.

One member of Recovery 2-Day™ was living in his car when he sought help. After detox, he continued to live in his car, while he found a job and saved enough money to move out of his car. Eventually, this same man who suffered lost love and learned the hard lessons of the defensive prayer, is now engaged to be married. He works in the treatment-therapy industry, helping men and women get well.

It is wise that women guide women and men guide men. It is wise for women to start women's groups, since they need to bond and seek the security women can offer each other. Many meetings historically have been breeding grounds for lonely hearts groups. But people come here for help, not sex. Sadly, often women who enter meeting rooms are attacked with sexual advances the moment they appear. Being married does not stop the advances, either.

These women are coming for help, respect them, and let them get well. The same is true of our male members, and it's important to let them get well before forming romantic relationships.

We have women in Recovery 2-Day™, we have men in Recovery 2-Day™. Treat them with the respect they deserve.

If you are asked to be a guide,
do the right thing
and set a good example for others.